HEALTH RECOVERY SECRETS

**A Revolutionary Guide To
Natural Healing & Self-Control**

DOUGLAS J. ELLISON

HEALTH RECOVERY SECRETS
A Revolutionary Guide To
Natural Healing & Self-Control

ISBN: 978-1532796449

Printed in the United States of America

DEDICATION

To God,
and my grandchildren,
Ty, Jade and Troy.

ACKNOWLEDGEMENT

I would like to thank Dr. Robert S. Mendelsohn, Dr. Robert C. Atkins, Dr. Tullio Simoncini, Dr. Paavo Airola, Dr. Maxwell Maltz, Dr. Otto Warburg, Dr. Linus Pauling, Suzanne Somers, Jack Lalanne, Henry Ford, Thomas Edison, John F. Kennedy and the other people mentioned in this book. Your stories or quotes helped make this book possible.

I also want to give a special thank you to Bonnie Cheney, Jamey Herzer, Terry McConnell, Michael Anderson and my daughter Genna Romero.

DISCLAIMER

INTRODUCTION

Health Recovery Secrets is a revolutionary course in natural healthcare. It's a simple, scientific and effective method for changing your habits and health. It contains powerful and easy to understand knowledge that will show you how to take care of your body and develop self-control. As you take more control of your thoughts, emotions and behavior you will change your life.

You will discover the secrets of how to prevent and recover from cancer, diabetes, heart disease, AIDS and many other chronic diseases and mental disorders. This knowledge will help you decide when you need a doctor, and when it's better to take care of yourself.

To get the most out of this book, I recommend keeping a dictionary by your side. If you don't understand the meaning of any word, it's best not to continue reading until you do understand. I also recommend doing your own research.

This workbook is meant to be examined carefully, not merely read once for entertainment. You'll remember more and develop greater understanding each time you read it. As you practice each exercise, you will develop new beliefs and habits.

It usually takes at least 21 days to gradually create a new habit or let go of an old one. Some beliefs are slow to change, while others can be changed in seconds.

Health Recovery Secrets will be your guide, so refer back to it often, in the same way an auto mechanic would use a manual to care for and repair an automobile.

CONTENTS

SECTION 3 HOW TO DEVELOP SELF-CONTROL

SECTION ONE

Healthcare Secrets

"For the great enemy of the truth
is very often not the lie...
deliberate, contrived and dishonest...
but the myth...
persistent, pervasive and unrealistic."

- President John F. Kennedy

IMPORTANT DEFINITIONS

Disease:
illness, imbalance or a destructive
process in an organism

Disorder:
illness, a lack of order or confusion

Myth:
any fictitious story, person, or thing

Theory:
a formulation of principles which have not
been proven completely; a speculation,
conjecture or guess

CHAPTER ONE

Empower Yourself

"The natural desire of good men is knowledge."
-Leonardo da Vinci

As you read this book you will be empowering yourself. You will learn secret knowledge and natural cures for many chronic diseases. You will also discover how to create a healthy body and develop more self-control.

MEDICAL TRAINING AND DRUG COMPANIES

"Only approximately six percent of the graduating
physicians in the U.S. have any training in nutrition."
-Ray D. Strand,M.D.

Knowledge is power. Whoever controls the medical textbooks, controls the physician's minds. If they believe they have been taught the truth, they won't seek to discover the truth.

Drug companies fund many major universities. They influence the school curriculum and the information put in medical textbooks. Most physicians have little or no training in nutrition and proper care of the human body.

Many textbooks contain myths and theories which are presented as proven facts. The lack of correct information in medical textbooks makes solving health problems harder, if not impossible. Vital knowledge is being suppressed.

The *Merck Manual* is the world's most widely used medical textbook for diagnosing and treating diseases. It has been used by doctors since it was first published in 1899. **The *Merck Manual* is published by Merck & Company, one of the largest drug manufacturers on earth.**

Pharmaceutical companies are in the business of selling patented products. One reason why drug companies discourage natural healing with healthy foods is they cannot be patented. Drug companies want to increase their profits by developing and selling more drugs.

"All drug companies in the U.S. are controlled by the Rockefellers." -Eustace Mullins, Murder by Injection

SYMPTOMS AND DISEASES

When doctors diagnose patients, they look for symptoms. The symptoms are then given disease names. Many times, physicians don't know what is causing their patient's bodies to malfunction. They often treat them with prescription drugs or surgery because that is what they have been trained to do.

Most medical research money is spent on everything but finding and scientifically proving the root cause of chronic diseases. Research results are often discarded or selected to support the point of view of their sponsors.

"Total U.S. spending on medical research has doubled in the past decade to nearly $95 billion a year."
-Associated Press, 2005

PRESCRIPTION DRUGS

"Some drugs must be used despite their having a very narrow margin of safety. There has always been a dark side to the discovery and use of drugs." -Merck Manual

Medical doctors use the *Physician's Desk Reference* and drug salesmen to learn about prescription drugs. **The PDR is published and controlled by drug companies.**
Most medicines, including over the counter painkillers, can cause side effects and death because they are poisonous.
Penicillin is a good example of a dangerous medicine. Penicillin is a powerful poison excreted by yeast. Antibiotics kill bad bacteria, but they also kill beneficial bacteria and white blood cells. Penicillin can save lives, but it can also cause fungal infections and death.
Television commercials are used to advertise drugs. The commercials disclose horrible side effects which are often worse than the symptoms they are supposed to control. **The third leading cause of death in the U.S. is conventional medical treatments, which includes prescription drugs.**

"The first duties of the physician is to educate the masses not to take medicine." -Dr. William Osler (1849-1919)
Founder of John Hopkins Hospital

3

U.S. FOOD AND DRUG ADMINISTRATION

The U.S. Food & Drug Administration has approved thousands of toxic substances. Some drugs are taken off the market after they have injured or killed many people. Drugs which cause milder side effects continue to be used.

Each new drug is supposed to be tested and proven to be safe and effective. Prescription medicines are one of the leading causes of addiction and death in the U.S.

The food and water most people are ingesting are poisoned with man-made chemicals, which have been approved by the FDA.

AMERICAN MEDICAL ASSOCIATION

"The AMA is not opposed to smoking and tobacco."
-Edward Annis, President of the AMA, 1963-1964

The American Medical Association is the largest association of physicians in the U.S. It controls standards of training, education and practice of doctors.

In the 1960s cigarette commercials were on television. During this time, many doctors and the AMA endorsed smoking and opposed the Surgeon General's health warning on cigarette packs. At that time smoking was believed to be healthy, unless you smoked excessively.

The AMA and the Journal of the AMA don't have all the answers. Medicine is a confusing and complex science. Many physicians are misinformed by the AMA.

4

AMERICAN CANCER SOCIETY

"We know that cancer is one of the most preventable and most curable diseases." -American Cancer Society

Why do over 500,000 Americans die each year from one of the most preventable and most curable diseases? The American Cancer Society knows that good nutrition helps to prevent and cure cancer. Why doesn't the ACS focus on cancer prevention education? Commercials and school programs would help save thousands of lives each year.

Instead of promoting prevention information, they focus on soliciting donations, research and early detection exams. Early detection exams don't prevent cancer.

In 2014 the ACS spent approximately $600 million on cancer research. The money was used for prevention, genetic and drug research.

"Everyone should know most cancer research is a fraud." -Dr. Linus Pauling, two-time Nobel Prize winner

CHRONIC DISEASES

Chronic diseases are the leading cause of death in the U.S. 133 million Americans have at least one chronic disease, such as heart disease, asthma, diabetes and cancer.

Millions of Americans die each year from chronic diseases caused by poisons, processed foods and fungal infections. The symptoms they cause are given many different disease names.

"U.S. Annual Healthcare Spending is a
Stunning $3.4 Trillion" *-Forbes magazine, 2014*

HEALTHCARE CHOICES

"The only real security that a man can have in this
world is a reserve of knowledge, experience and ability."
-Henry Ford

Healthcare isn't designed to be affordable. It's designed to be profitable. Doctors, nurses and scientists don't have all the answers and drug companies are misinforming them.

Conventional and alternative healthcare are imperfect. Some elements of each type of healthcare are good, while others are harmful. Integrative healthcare often combines the use of nutrition and poisonous chemicals.

Health Recovery Secrets will empower you with vital knowledge so you can take more control of your mental and physical health. It will help you decide when you need a doctor, and when it's better to care for yourself.

"A desire to be in charge of our own lives,
a need for control, is born in each of us.
It is essential to our mental health,
and our success, that we take control."
-Robert Foster Bennett

*"Never let formal education
get in the way of your learning."*
-*Mark Twain*

SUMMARY

1. The *Merck Manual* is the world's most widely used medical textbook for diagnosing and treating diseases. It's controlled and published by a drug manufacturer.
2. Drug companies manipulate the information in many medical textbooks. The lack of correct knowledge in textbooks makes solving health problems harder, if not impossible.
3. Most physicians aren't trained to prevent and heal chronic diseases using nutrition. They are trained to use drugs, surgery and other expensive procedures.
4. Conventional and alternative healthcare are imperfect. Medicine isn't an exact science. Some elements of each type of healthcare are good, while others are harmful.
5. Millions of Americans have chronic pain and disease symptoms caused by poisons, which have been approved by the FDA.
6. Some statistics, research, associations and government agencies misinform us.
7. Millions of Americans die each year from chronic diseases caused by poisons, processed foods and fungal infections.
8. Empower yourself with more knowledge.

"Any breakthrough in science is likely to come from outside the system. Experts are the most familiar with the developed knowledge inside the prescribed boundaries of a given science."

-Maxwell Maltz, M.D.

CHAPTER TWO

Cancer Secrets

"No one knows the exact cause of most cases of cancer.
We now know that some cancers are caused by infections."
-American Cancer Society

I know a man named Bob. He developed skin cancer. Bob had a procedure done to remove the growth from his nose. A few months later, the growth returned. His doctor then told Bob he didn't get all of the cancer cells and needed to operate again. He said, "I need to remove most of your nose to get all of the cancer."

Bob refused to have the procedure done and he told the doctor, "I would rather die than walk around without a nose."

Then the strangest thing happened. The doctor suggested he try an antifungal cream on his nose. Bob used the cream and within a few weeks, his cancer was gone.

How could an antifungal cream kill cancer cells? Bob believed, like most oncologists, that cancer cells are mutated human cells.

"Cancer is one hundred times more likely to occur in people
who take drugs that suppress the immune system."
-Merck Medical Manual

I met a man named Don. He eventually died from cancer. Don told me he went to the doctor because he had a lung infection. The doctor told him his white blood cells were attacking him. His doctor then prescribed chemotherapy drugs to suppress his immune system.

Don's immune system gradually became weaker each day. He eventually needed an oxygen tank to breathe. When Don returned to the doctor for more tests, he was told he had fungus in his liver. A couple of days later, he received a phone call from his doctor. His doctor told him he had misdiagnosed him. Don was told he had cancer of the liver and was prescribed more chemotherapy pills.

The chemicals further suppressed his immune system. Don died after months of chemical poisoning. His body could no longer fight the cancer cells without healthy white blood cells.

Is it possible the cells attacking Don's lungs and liver were fungus and not white blood cells? Is it also possible his doctor was correct when he told Don he had fungus in his liver? I believe chemotherapy and fungus killed Don.

KNOCKOUT CANCER

Suzanne Somers wrote a book called, *Knockout*. In her book she tells her personal story of being diagnosed with cancer. She went to the hospital because she developed welts, a rash and difficulty breathing. Her doctors gave her a CT scan before telling her she had cancerous tumors and a blood clot.

Her physicians were convinced Suzanne had cancer. She wasn't convinced, so she requested a biopsy to check for fungus. She believed she may have contracted valley fever.

When the results of the biopsy came back, the pathologist told her she had a fungal infection. Suzanne was then told she had leprosy, tuberculosis or valley fever.

Suzanne refused chemotherapy and other poisonous drugs. She didn't blindly believe the doctors and allow them to scare her into treatments which would weaken her body and possibly kill her.

Suzanne almost died from the powerful toxins the fungi excreted in her body. The CT scan and biopsy *proved* fungus can create tumors and white clots. Her experience also *proved* how little oncologists and pathologists know about fungal infections.

Suzanne Somers wasn't misdiagnosed with cancer. She did have a type of cancer. Cancer cells are fungus cells. **The oncologists and the pathologist were both correct.**

CANCER TUMORS

Cancer is a disease which kills over eight million men, women and children worldwide every year. According to the World Health Organization, cancer is a leading cause of death.

The conventional definition of cancer is a malignant tumor which can spread. Cancer cells are considered abnormal cells which grow out of control, invade and attack the body. Cancer cells can do things which are **impossible** for human cells to do, such as live without oxygen.

Cancer is a disease caused by uncontrolled fungus cells which spread and destroy healthy body tissues.

Webster's dictionary defines a tumor as an abnormal growth of new tissue, independent of its surrounding structure. The key word is independent. **Cancer growths are the body of colonizing fungi, called mycelium.**

"Fungi are everywhere. There are approximately 1.5 million species of fungi on earth, but only about 300 of those are known to make people sick." -Center for Disease Control

Fungal growths are given different names depending on their appearance and the part of the body they are found. There are about 300 different species of fungi which cause human illnesses.

Cancer tumors, fibroids, psoriasis, sclerosis, cirrhosis, polyps, plaques, goiters, thrombus, white blood clots, warts and moles are fungal growths.

Doctors classify fungal tumors as benign, until the slow growing tumors begin to grow quickly or they spread. Some oncologists call benign tumors precancerous growths because they are likely to become cancerous. Moles are a good example of fungal growths that are called cancerous tumors (melanomas) when they begin to grow quickly.

A friend of mine, named Bonnie developed a fungal growth on her thyroid. Her doctor called it a goiter. She was told her growth was caused by a malfunctioning thyroid. Bonnie had the tumor surgically removed. The surgeon removed 75% of her thyroid to get most of the fungus cells.

She now takes natural dried pig thyroid daily. Synthetic thyroid is poisonous and causes many side effects. Her growth was classified as non-cancerous because it was slow growing and hadn't spread.

The actress Mary Tyler Moore developed a brain tumor. The fungal growth eventually wrapped around her optic nerve, so she had surgery to remove it. Because the tumor was slow growing and hadn't spread to other parts of the body, it was classified as non-cancerous.

AIDS

"AIDS: a condition of deficiency of certain leukocytes, resulting in infections, cancer, neural degeneration, etc."
-Webster's New World Dictionary

People with cancer also suffer from a condition called AIDS. The acronym AIDS stands for Acquired Immune Deficiency Syndrome. AIDS is a condition in which a person has a deficiency of healthy white blood cells (leukocytes) and becomes less able to control fungus and bacteria.

Poisonous man-made chemicals and drugs compromise the immune system. **The end result is a deficiency of white blood cells and fungal infections, such as cancer.**

"Fungi have a special tendency to cause infections in people with a compromised immune system."
-Merck Medical Manual

There are degrees in the deficiency of white blood cells. Whenever a person is poisoned, some white blood cells and beneficial bacteria are destroyed. Red (oxygen) blood cells are also damaged, which causes a low oxygen bloodstream and then fungi begin to ferment, spread and create tumors.

13

"Research has shown that the longer and more intensely the immune system is suppressed...the higher the risk of cancer."
-American Cancer Society

A deficiency of red and white blood cells can be a chronic condition caused by the many poisons in the air, food and water. **Chemotherapy is a great example of how chemical poisoning causes AIDS.**

Damaged human cells never invade and attack other human cells. When human cells are damaged, they mutate, become weaker and die. Leukemia and many other autoimmune disorders are caused by fungus and the toxins they excrete.

The greatest myth about human cancer cells
is, they are mutated or immature human cells.

CANCER CELLS ARE ANAEROBIC CELLS

"Cancer cells are anaerobic and have the ability to ferment. All human cells have an absolute requirement for oxygen, but cancer cells can live without oxygen a rule without exception." *-Dr. Otto Warburg, Nobel Prize winner*

Dr. Warburg was talking about the fact that cancer cells are anaerobic cells and they can live without oxygen by fermenting. Human cells are aerobic cells and must have oxygen because they cannot ferment. If you don't believe human cells must have oxygen, tie a tourniquet around any part of your body to test the theory.

In 1838, pathologist Johannes Muller discovered cancer cells were not human cells and they were developed by *budding organisms.*

14

Dr. Tullio Simoncini, is an Italian oncologist. He believes cancer cells are fungus cells. He also believes Candida albicans is one type of fungus which causes cancerous tumors. He discovered that every cancerous tumor he examined under a microscope, was made of fungus cells. Dr. Simoncini has successfully used bicarbonate of soda to eliminate cancer cells. His website is **cancerisafungus.com**

Many cancer patients undergoing chemotherapy die from chemical poisoning and an infestation of fungus.

HELA CELLS ARE FUNGUS CELLS

The word Hela is an abbreviation for Henrietta Lacks. In 1951, George Gey took what was believed to be mutated human cancer cells from Henrietta Lacks, who died from cervical cancer.

Over 70,000 articles have been written about Hela cells. Hela cells have been used in cancer research worldwide for over 60 years. They are believed to be the only immortal human cells. **All other attempts to grow human cells outside the body have failed because Hela cells are actually fungus cells. Scientists are unaware of this big misunderstanding.**

"In the spring of 1953, a cell culture factory was established at Tuskegee University to supply Jonas Salk, as well as other labs, with Hela cells. Less than a year later Salk's vaccine was ready for human trials." -Wikipedia

Some fungus cells reproduce using the fission method like human cells. Many types of fungus cells look similar to human cells, while others look like rod shaped bacteria.

15

Fungus and human cells are eukaryotic cells. They both have a nucleus, cholesterol and DNA. Bacteria cells are prokaryotic cells. They don't have a nucleus.

Scientists use yeast in lab experiments worldwide because they grow much faster than human cells. Yeast is the model organism used in cell research. They are easily kept alive in laboratories and used to test the toxicity of new drugs.

Fungus spores are seeds which can lay dormant for years in the soil or the human body. When the environment is right they germinate and grow.

"Unlike normal cells, cancer cells are often very different in their size and shape." -American Cancer Society

Ten Reasons Why Cancer Cells Are Fungus Cells

1. Cancer and some fungus are facultative anaerobic cells. They can live with or without oxygen. Human cells are aerobic cells which die when deprived of oxygen.
2. Cancer and fungus can ferment. Human cells can't ferment.
3. Cancer and fungus cells can multiply much faster than human cells.
4. Cancer and fungus have a larger nucleus and more chromosomes than human cells.
5. Cancer cells and fungus grow and spread like parasites.
6. Cancer and fungus cells can attach and hide within human tissues, including bones.

7. Cancer and fungus can colonize and create tumors.
8. Cancer and fungus have a hard cell wall. Human cells don't.
9. Cancer and fungus thrive on acidic refined sugars and grains.
10. Cancer and fungus are considered immortal cells. They aren't actually immortal. The original cells die, but their offspring continue to reproduce.

"Breast cancer cells can spread by breaking away from a tumor. They can travel through the blood. After spreading cancer cells may attach to other tissues and grow to form new tumors." -National Cancer Institute

FUNGUS AMONG US

Everyone has fungus cells in their body. Candida albicans is one type of fungus which normally lives in and on our bodies. Candida is a *beneficial* part of intestinal flora when the body is functioning properly.

Our bodies are hosts for many types of microbes. Some microorganisms are essential to the proper functioning of our bodies. Symbiosis is the living together of two kinds of organisms to their mutual advantage. Scientists recently discovered the importance of beneficial bacteria.

Candida will ferment and grow out of control when the bloodstream is low in oxygen and white blood cells. To prevent or stop fungal infections such as cancer, we need to avoid poisons and give our bodies the proper nutrients.

CONVENTIONAL CANCER TREATMENTS

*"Cancer is caused by carcinogens: radiation,
chemicals and germs." -World Health Organization*

Oncologists have been taught to fight cancer with surgery, chemotherapy, and radiation. All three methods weaken the immune system. Radiation and chemotherapy poison and kill red blood cells. They also destroy beneficial bacteria, and white blood cells which are needed to control the growth of harmful fungus and bacteria.

SURGERY

Surgery is a traumatic experience to the body. Over 400,000 patients in the U.S. die each year from complications caused by surgeon errors, anesthetics, medication and germs acquired while in the hospital.

Cancer surgery is sometimes necessary and life-saving. When it comes to eliminating most fungal growths, surgery should be one of your last choices. Systemic fungal infections cannot be stopped using surgery.

*"Modern cancer surgery will someday be regarded with the
same kind of horror that we now regard the use of leeches in
George Washington's time." -Dr. Robert Mendelsohn*

After surgery, the patient is in a weakened state. At that time, more antibiotics are usually given. If the infection is caused by bacteria, then antibiotics may help save the patient. When the infection is caused by fungus, antibiotics can help fungus grow and eventually kill the patient.

Surgery can help cancer cells spread, because surgery weakens the body. Anesthetics and antibiotics poison the bloodstream and create a deficiency of healthy white blood cells (AIDS).

RADIATION

"Cancer is caused by an agent called carcinogen such as a chemical, a virus, radiation or sunlight."
-Merck Manual

Radiologists know that some types of radiation damage cells. Radiation poisoning can cause AIDS and fungal infections in healthy people. **The Merck Manual believes cancer is caused by radiation, but still recommends using it to kill cancer cells.**

CHEMOTHERAPY

Chemotherapy is chemical poisoning. Many oncologists will not use this therapy when they develop cancer. They know poisons can cause AIDS and help cancer spread.

Chemical therapy kills fungus cells, but it also poisons the entire body. The poison destroys white blood cells and reduces the body's ability to create them again. Bones can become brittle and easily break. I know two women who suffered broken necks before dying of cancer.

Oncologists create the condition called AIDS before performing a bone marrow transplant. They deliberately kill the patient's white blood cells, because they believe immature white blood cells are attacking the body.

19

The patient may then die from complications created by suppressing the immune system. The complications are severe fungal infections or organ failure.

"Cancer is one hundred times more likely to occur in people who take drugs that suppress the immune system."
-Merck Manual

Oncologists believe cancer cells can become more aggressive and spread quickly after surgery, radiation or chemotherapy. What actually occurs is, patients become more deficient in white blood cells and beneficial bacteria, which are needed to control fungus. Now, the patients are almost defenseless.

Chemical poisoning may not kill all of the fungi and fungus spores before it kills the patient. As the spores germinate, the body will become infected again. Patients can also become infected with different types of bacteria or fungus in their weakened state.

ANTIFUNGAL DRUGS

Antifungals are poisonous and cause disease symptoms when taken orally. Cancer cells can be controlled by diet, herbs, baking soda and healthier methods.

Taking antifungal drugs orally has been known to cause organ failure and death. Some of the side effects are: kidney and liver failure, anemia, hearing loss, difficulty breathing, hepatitis, bone marrow suppression, deficiency of minerals, jaundice, fever and irregular heartbeat.

"Conventional medicine's approach to cancer prevention and treatment is a debilitating, often deadly fraud."

-*Suzanne Somers*

SUMMARY

1. Cancer cells are fungus cells.
2. AIDS is a deficiency of healthy white blood cells.
3. Vaccines, antibiotics, drugs and and other poisons cause AIDS and systemic fungal infections.
4. All cancer patients have a deficiency of white blood cells. There are degrees of AIDS.
5. Hela cells are fungus cells.
6. Fungus and human cells are eukaryotic cells. They contain a nucleus, cholesterol and DNA.
7. Cancer cells aren't immature or mutated cells.
8. Surgery, radiation and chemotherapy don't address the cause of systemic fungal infections.
9. Fungal infections cause many disease symptoms.
10. Radiation and chemotherapy can cause AIDS and cancer.

"The three great essentials to achieve anything worthwhile are: hard work, persistence and common sense."

"If we did all the things we are capable of, we would literally astound ourselves."

-Thomas Edison

CHAPTER THREE

Conquer Cancer

" Modern Medicine would rather you die using its remedies than live by using what physicians call quackery. "
-Dr. Robert Mendelsohn

Patrick Swayze was a well-known actor who died from cancer. He was diagnosed with cancer in 2008 and received 10 months of chemotherapy. Patrick was a positive thinker and a brave fighter, but he still died.

Muhammad Ali is known as one of the best fighters in boxing history. When he was a young man he had fast hands and feet. As he became older and slower, he changed his strategy of fighting. He lay on the ropes more and let his opponents punch him. The end result was brain damage, from the blows to his head. After each fight, Ali progressively talked and walked slower.

If you use conventional cancer treatments, you will be taking blows to your immune system. Surgery, radiation and chemotherapy are not the best strategies to control fungus cells.

Over 500,000 men, women and children die from cancer each year in the U.S. They die regardless of all the modern technology, chemotherapy drugs, surgery and radiation. **The right strategy is a vital key to becoming healthy again.**

MIND OVER MATTER

*"It's easier to fool people than to convince them
that they have been fooled." -Mark Twain*

Norman Cousins wrote a book called, *Anatomy of an Illness.* In his book, he tells the story of how he became seriously ill and then well again. It's a myth Norman Cousins healed himself by using mind over matter and funny movies. **Norman avoided hospitals and prescription drugs.** He began receiving large doses of vitamin C intravenously every day. Norman did succeed in cleansing his body of heavy metals and other poisons. He also gave his body the nutrients it needed to become healthy again. **Norman Cousins used the right strategy and took aggressive action.**

If you are suffering from cancer, heart disease, or diabetes, I don't recommend ignoring your problem by watching funny movies or telling yourself the problem isn't as bad as it really is. Laughter can help release tension, but it's not enough.

Many positive thinking people deny reality. There are a lot of people who have died while visualizing their white blood cells beating up cancer cells. Positive thinking can have a negative effect when it's unrealistic.

Many people deceive themselves with positive thinking. They die from drugs, diseases or dangerous activities while believing they will not.

Emile Coue said, "Always think of what you have to do as easy and it will become so." Is this realistic thinking? Aren't some things hard to do regardless of what you think? Coue also said, "Every day in every way I'm getting better and better." Is this positive affirmation realistic? Is it the way to solve real life problems?

Napoleon Hill said, "Whatever the mind of man can conceive and believe it can achieve." Is that quote realistic thinking? Aren't mental hospitals full of people who conceive and believe irrational ideas?

Scientists and doctors believe many unproven and unrealistic theories. Sometimes the minds of men are deceived by the ideas they have conceived and believed.

Many people become mentally defeated when their doctor tells them they have an incurable disease and are going to die. Because they believe the doctor's words, they don't seek alternative knowledge which could heal them. They give up because they believe it's hopeless

Some people seem to want to die. They may be slowly killing themselves with processed foods and drugs long before they develop cancer.

Positive thinking can help, but it's not enough. A person must want to live and become determined to find out what they must do to get well. We need correct knowledge and the right strategy to succeed. Then we must take aggressive action until we become healthy.

HEALTHY CHOICES

It's almost impossible to make good choices without correct knowledge. I believe most people eat unhealthy foods, because they taste good or make them feel good. Many people don't realize how unhealthy some processed foods really are.

Some people believe when they become ill, doctors can solve their health problems with a pill. Disease symptoms aren't caused by a deficiency of prescription drugs.

This book was written to help you become healthy without expensive conventional or alternative treatments. Americans spend over $30 billion a year on alternative healthcare products and services. Some of them are ineffective and give false hope.

Your body needs whole organic food and clean water. As long as your diet includes a lot of poisoned and mineral deficient food, don't expect to be healthy.

These alternative treatments will help your body eliminate and control fungus, without killing white blood cells.

ALTERNATIVE CANCER TREATMENTS

1. Massage, acupuncture and chiropractic therapies can help relieve pain, tension and correct some injuries. They can't cure cancer and most chronic degenerative diseases which are caused by poisons and fungal infections.

2. Immunotherapy is not recommended. The use of man-made chemicals to induce, enhance or suppress the immune system are unnecessary and can be harmful.

3. Gene targeted therapy is not recommended. This therapy is based on the theory that cancer cells are human cells and a genetic problem. This therapy can cost over $30,000 a month.

4. Carrot juice and coffee enema therapy is not recommended. This therapy may also include the use of antibiotics which help cancer cells grow. The caffeine in coffee is poison. Enemas should be done using pure warm water. If you suffer from blood sugar imbalances like diabetes or hypoglycemia, carrot juice (high in sugar) and caffeine can slow down the healing process.

Green vegetable juices and pure water enemas help speed up the healing process by alkalizing, cleansing and giving the body essential nutrients. You can recover your health without juicing. It will take longer.

5. Laetrile therapy is not needed. Cancer cells aren't mutated human cells which lack cyanide (B17).

6. Vitamin C therapy can be helpful. Taking ascorbic acid pills or injections will help to cleanse the body of microbes and poisons. It's best to eat raw organic fruits and vegetables, and drink fresh vegetable juices to get vitamin C and other essential nutrients.

7. Oxygen (Ozone) therapy can be helpful, but it's not needed to regain your health. Facultative bacteria and fungus can live with or without oxygen, while white blood cells must have oxygen. Exercise, deep breathing and clean water supply oxygen. Poisons in food and water cause low oxygen in the bloodstream by killing red blood cells.

8. Colloidal silver and gold can be helpful. I believe diet and powerful herbs are more effective for controlling microbes, detoxing and supplying needed nutrients.

9. Green juice therapy can help tremendously. Fresh, organic green vegetables supply chlorophyll and other nutrients the body needs to operate properly. Wheat grass can be healthy, unless the wheat has been poisoned with pesticides. Cilantro, romaine lettuce, cucumbers and kale are great for alkalizing the body.

Juice therapy can help alcoholics and other drug users to detox in a less painful way. Most alcoholics lack essential minerals and suffer from hypoglycemia. Juicing supplies large amounts of vitamins, minerals and other nutrients. Green juice fasting for 3 days can be helpful, but it's not necessary to regain health. Green juices help speed up the healing process.

Adding psyllium husks to your diet is also helpful for detoxing the body. The husks add fiber which helps to clean the intestines and remove toxins. Constipation can cause illness and death.

10. Water fasting is a great way to flush out toxins and help kill germs. The body can store harmful substances. When you don't eat, your body will begin a cleansing process. Water is one of the best ways to cleanse your body and supply alkalizing minerals. I recommend drinking 4 or more 16 ounce glasses of clean water every day. Fasting helps speed up the healing process. Overeating is an unhealthy habit.

11. Sauna therapy helps to detox the body and kill fungus. As you create an artificial fever, you sweat out toxins and the higher temperature kills germs. Mineral hot springs have been used for hundreds of years to help heal the body. You should drink more water to avoid dehydration and supply needed minerals lost from sweating.

12. Homeopathic and Naturopathic medicine are not recommended. Both are unnecessary and can be harmful.

13. Niacin therapy works well with sauna therapy to flush out toxins. 100 milligrams of flushing niacin per day helps to remove harmful substances in the body. Flushing niacin taken in larger amounts has been successfully used to detox drug residue.

14. Herbal tea therapy is one of the fastest and most effective ways to help alkalize the bloodstream, control fungus and flush out toxins. This therapy combines the use of water and healing herbs. The best tea on the market is **Cellular Tea.** This tea contains many of the most powerful herbs available and has been used successfully to eliminate cancer tumors. Cellular Tea is a beneficial daily supplement and is sold online @ **cellulartea.com**

Ojibwa tea has been used successfully to kill fungus and other pathogens for many years. Ojibwa tea contains burdock root, Indian-rhubarb root, sheep sorrel and slippery elm. Herbal remedies are the most effective when you stop poisoning your body with processed foods. Herbs contain many healthy nutrients.

Herbal cleansing formulas which come in capsule form help to cleanse the body of toxins and harmful germs. The dried herbs must be taken in concentration to be effective.

15. **Four Thieves Vinegar** was originally used by grave robbers to kill germs and stay healthy during the Black Plague. It is a blend of apple cider vinegar, garlic, thyme, rosemary and other herbs.

16. **Garlic** has been used by people to kill pathogens for thousands of years. It can be used topically as an antibiotic.

"Garlic extract stops plaque buildup in arteries."
-David Eifrig, M.D.

17. **Cold pressed, organic olive oil** is a powerful germ killer. Olive oil can be used for ear infections. Warm olive oil in the ear helps kill bacteria and fungus. Olive oil can also be used to help dissolve and purge liver, kidney and gall bladder stones. Olive oil, apple cider vinegar and raw honey make a healthy salad dressing.

18. **Apples and unpasteurized apple cider vinegar** are natural germ fighters. They contain sulfur, potassium, enzymes, beneficial bacteria and alkalizing minerals. Two or more tablespoons of organic raw apple cider vinegar, with raw honey, in a glass of clean water is an excellent daily supplement.

Eating an organic apple a day is better for you than synthetic vitamin-mineral pills. You may want to peel them because some apples have a coating of wax applied to them.

19. Baking soda neutralizes poisons, alkalizes blood, and helps kill germs. The pancreas naturally creates sodium bicarbonate to alkalize the body. When the pancreas is malfunctioning or overwhelmed, your body becomes very acidic. Refined sugars and grains are two main causes of acidosis.

Baking soda is only a temporary fix. You want to alkalize and hydrate your body with clean water, raw whole foods and green juices.

This is a quick method to control fungus and neutralize poisons.

Step one. Stop eating dead foods, especially refined sugars, grains and processed meats.

Step two. Drink a 16 ounce glass of clean water with one tablespoon of baking soda three times per day between meals.

Step three. Continue the baking soda treatment 7 days in a row. Then use baking soda every other 7 days, until the fungus is under control.

Baking soda can be used as toothpaste and an antacid.

Baking soda and water will neutralize the oils from poison oak and ivy. Baking soda paste can also be used on bites and stings from spiders, snakes and bees to stop pain and cell damage.

Drinking baking soda will help neutralize the injected venom. Take one tablespoon of baking soda with a 16 ounce glass of water every hour, up to 6 times per day. Continue until the poisons are neutralized.

Antivenoms are often ineffective, expensive and can cause severe side effects. Many times survival depends on the toxicity of the venom, how much was injected and how well the person or animal can tolerate the poison until it's neutralized.

20. Probiotics are supplements made of beneficial bacteria. They help replace bacteria which is killed when eating processed foods, using antibiotics and other drugs. The best way to replenish good bacteria is by eating organic fruits, vegetables and green drinks. Organic raw apple cider vinegar and healthy fermented foods also have beneficial bacteria.

21. Hydrogen Peroxide can be used to kill fungal and bacterial growths on the skin. It can be purchased at the store in 3% form or food grade 35% at some health food stores.

Hydrogen Peroxide is used in many skin care products and is the same substance used by white blood cells to kill germs and neutralize poisons. The 3% hydrogen peroxide can also be used to whiten teeth.

22. Salicylic acid is sold at pharmacies. The 17% acid solution comes in a liquid form. It can be used to remove corns, warts. moles, age spots, and other fungal growths without damaging the skin.

To remove fungus growths on the skin apply 17% salicylic acid on the growth once a day. Peel off the white film after 8 hours. Don't try to scrape off the growth. Let the acid gradually remove it. Use the acid every day for up to one week. Then use salicylic acid every other week until the fungal growths are eliminated.

Salicylic acid is used in many anti-acne and psoriasis skin products in a 2% cream solution. It will kill the bacteria and fungus which cause acne and psoriasis. When used topically it is effective and safe. Avoid eye contact.

Aspirin pills are a form of salicylic acid. Salicylic acid is poisonous and can be harmful when taken orally. Aspirin taken in large amounts will cause thin blood, internal bleeding and death.

23. Antibiotic creams, when used topically for skin or ear infections can be effective and safe. If an ear infection is caused by bacteria, then antibiotic ointment can be effective when packed inside the ear. Antibiotics, when taken orally, are known to cause fungal infections and destroy beneficial bacteria.

24. Ultraviolet light therapy can help control toenail fungus. Toenail fungus thrives on refined sugars and grains. There are laser nail fungus therapies that cost hundreds to thousands of dollars. The UV lamps used to cure nail polish generate the same UV-A light as laser therapy or sunlight. You will want to file down your nails to help the ultraviolet light penetrate. Use the lamp 15-30 minutes per day. The fungus can return if you eat sugary foods which feed it.

25. Vitamin D therapy will help control cancer cells. Our bodies require sunlight to create Vitamin D. A lack of this hormone has been linked to cancer, asthma and other fungal infections. Sunbathing or Vitamin D3 supplements will help create a stronger immune system.

"Vitamin D, a steroid hormone that influences virtually every cell in your body, is easily one of nature's most potent cancer fighters."
-Dr. Joseph Mercola

"Our greatest weakness lies in giving up.
The most certain way to succeed is always to try
just one more time." -Thomas A. Edison

SUMMARY

1. Most alternative treatments and supplements are unnecessary if you eat mainly whole, organic foods and drink clean water. Poisons and mineral deficiencies are two of the main causes of systemic fungal infections and chronic disease symptoms.
2. Herbs help white blood cells kill pathogens and cleanse the blood. Garlic, apples and apple cider vinegar all help the body control germs.
3. Enemas using warm pure water can help cleanse the body of poisons faster than diet alone. Water fasting helps detox the body.
4. Green vegetable juicing is a good method for alkalizing the blood and supplying essential nutrients the body may be lacking. Juicing is superior to synthetic vitamin-mineral supplements.
5. Baking soda helps neutralize poisons and control germs.
6. Hydrogen peroxide and salicylic acid can be used to solve many skin problems.
7. Lots of rest and clean water are two of the best ways to help your body get well. Relax and use all of your energy to detox and kill germs.
8. Changing your diet will change your life.
9. Start taking action to create a healthy body.

*"Viruses are identified by
the type of changes
they cause in the cell."*

-American Cancer Society

CHAPTER FOUR

Virus Secrets

*"Viruses cannot be identified using a microscope
because they are too small." -Merck Manual*

Viruses aren't identified in the same way as bacteria and
fungus because they are poisons, not living cells. Many
viruses are never actually identified. The symptoms they cause
are given disease names such as polio, herpes, chicken pox,
shingles, smallpox, rabies, ebola, influenza, cold, malaria,
yellow fever and HIV.

*"Virus [Latin, a poison] a microscopic
infectious agent causing various diseases."*
- Webster's New World Dictionary, 2006

Virus is the Latin word for poison. Some viruses contain
DNA. DNA is nucleic acid. It's found in the cells of people
and fungus. These acid molecules are also found in human
feces and feces excreted by fungus. Fungus cells excrete
viruses that contain DNA.

The science of virology is based on many unproven
theories and wrong conclusions. Scientists can't decide what
viruses are.

"For about 100 years, the scientific community repeatedly changed its collective mind over what viruses are. First seen as poisons, then as life forms, then biological chemicals."
-Dr. Luis Villarreal, virologist, UC Irvine

Viruses are not living cells like fungus and bacteria. They don't have cell walls because they are not cells. The belief that non-living substances can incubate or replicate is a myth.

"Despite his other successes Louis Pasteur (1822-1895) was unable to find the causative agent for rabies and speculated about a pathogen too small to be detected using a microscope." -Wikipedia

FUNGUS POISONS

There are about 300 species of fungi which cause human illness. Aspergillus, cryptococcus, candida albicans, penicillium, and others excrete viruses. Symptoms caused by fungal excrements are often classified as viral infections and diseases.

Penicillium is the type of fungus used to create the virus called penicillin. Penicillin has been used to save lives. It also causes fungal infections and kills beneficial bacteria, and human cells.

"Microorganisms are a leading cause of death in the world."
-World Health Organization

How do vaccine makers grow viruses if they aren't alive? They grow fungus and bacteria in their germ factories, like the one established in 1953, at Tuskegee University. Then they harvest the viruses that the fungus and bacteria excrete.

36

GENETICALLY MODIFIED ORGANISMS

Genetically modified organisms are plants, animals and microorganisms that have had their genetic material altered using genetic engineering techniques. Genetically modified microbes and the viruses they excrete can enter our bodies by way of food, water, vaccines, blood transfusions and other methods.

ANTIGENS

"Viruses also cause infections, but are too primitive to be classified as living organisms."
-Department of Health and Human Services

An antigen is any microbe or substance that causes your white blood cells to release antibodies to kill or neutralize it. Antigens infect and destroy living cells.

The definition of the word infect is to contaminate or cause to become diseased by contact with a disease producing *organism or substance.*

Infections can be caused by poisonous substances excreted by bacteria, fungus and parasites. After a microbe or parasite enters the body they begin damaging human cells, as they grow and excrete toxins.

Some of the deadliest viruses found in nature are excreted by fungus and bacteria. Prion is another name for poison.

Many antibiotics are made of fungus toxins. Erythromycin is made of ergot toxins. Ergotism is a good example of the powerful effects caused by a fungus virus.

Ergot fungus growing on rye grain killed thousands of people in the middle ages. It was known as Saint Anthony's fire because of the inflammation and burning sensation created by the fungal virus.

Poisons kill blood cells and beneficial bacteria, causing digestive problems. They can cause disease symptoms, such as inflammation, convulsions, anxiety, psychosis, headache, fever, swollen lymph nodes and tonsils, gangrene, paralysis, encephalitis, pox, nausea, vomiting, diarrhea, rashes and death. These symptoms have been given viral disease names such as polio, influenza, smallpox and rabies.

Botulism is a good example of how disease symptoms and even death are caused by bacterial viruses. Noroviruses are sometimes called food poisoning or the stomach flu.

Eating grains is a leading cause of food poisoning for cattle and human beings. Most commercially grown wheat, corn, oats, and soybeans are poisoned by fungus viruses, pesticides and other man-made chemicals. Some are GMOs.

"Virus classification is the subject of ongoing debate and proposals. This is mainly due to the pseudo-living nature of viruses, which is to say they are non-living particles."
-Wikipedia, Virus classification

MAN-MADE VIRUSES

Billions of people worldwide are being poisoned by man-made viruses. Chemical companies like Dow, Bayer and Monsanto are making huge profits while poisoning us.

Poisons are still poisons, even in small amounts. The fluoride put in city water and toothpaste is unhealthy. Each tube of toothpaste has a fluoride warning label on it because fluoride is a toxic substance.

Veterinarians are trained to promote vaccines and processed animal foods, which contain poisons. Many of them use the *Merck Veterinarian Manual* to diagnose and treat animal diseases. They are being deceived by drug and pet food companies. Wild animals have thrived for thousands of years without man-made vaccines and foods.

Many farmers use harmful chemicals when growing crops. These viruses end up in our soil, food and water. The farmers have been deceived by chemical companies.

FELINE LEUKEMIA VIRUS

"The cause of most types of leukemia isn't known. Viruses cause some leukemia in animals, such as cats."
-Merck Manual

Feline leukemia is caused by fungi and viruses. A cat's immune system can become compromised by man-made viruses in the food, water and vaccines. Fungus can then spread throughout the body and excrete their own viruses. The viruses infect the feline cells and cause them to mutate and die. The cancer cells are fungi cells, not mutated cat cells.

"Recently, there has been some controversy regarding duration of protection and timing of vaccination, as well as the safety and necessity of certain vaccines." - WebMD

EBOLA VIRUS

Information about the ebola virus causes confusion. Symptoms of the ebola virus are fever, dehydration, headache, muscle pain, weakness, fatigue, diarrhea, vomiting, abdominal pain, unexplained bleeding and death.

All these symptoms can be caused by poisons. Conventional healthcare has no specific treatment for the ebola virus, except water and I.V. fluids. Water and baking soda can be used to help neutralize and flush out this virus.

The ebola virus causes symptoms which are similar to aspirin. If you ingest too much aspirin, it causes brain damage, internal bleeding, and death.

Aspirin is a poison originally extracted from the bark of the willow tree. Millions of people have died from ingesting too much aspirin.

According to the *Merck Manual,* viruses cannot be identified using a microscope, yet there are images of a worm-like ebola virus on the Center for Disease Control website.

HUMAN PAPALLOMA VIRUS

Many doctors believe the human papalloma virus causes cervical cancer. Papalloma is another word for wart. Warts are fungal growths. The wart doesn't cause cancer, it is cancer. The virus is excreted by the fungus. The HPV vaccine contains fungi and poisons which cause infections, and sometimes sterility or death.

HUMAN IMMUNODEFICIENCY VIRUS

Many people diagnosed with HIV don't develop AIDS. HIV is not AIDS. AIDS is a deficiency of healthy white blood cells.

Tests used to identify HIV are not accurate. HIV cannot be identified with a microscope or a white blood cell count. Most viruses are never actually identified.

Some drugs used to treat HIV can cause life threatening side effects. The earliest drugs such as AZT were highly toxic and often caused AIDS and death.

Sexually transmitted diseases are caused by bacteria, fungus and parasites. The viruses they excrete can cause AIDS.

Many Africans die of AIDS because of starvation. Their lack of essential nutrients cause a deficiency of white blood cells, which results in infections and eventually death.

According to the CDC, the average annual cost of HIV care was $23,000 and lifetime treatment costs was $379,668 in 2010.

DARK FIELD MICROSCOPY

"Syphilis is what made dark field microscopy popular."
-C. Robert Bagnell, Jr. PhD., University of N.C.

Dark field microscopy is a type of light microscopy that produces brightly illuminated objects on a dark background. Syphilis was discovered in 1905 using a dark field microscope.

41

Today, dark field microscopy is considered quackery by many pathologists. Why is this, when dark field microscopy was proven so successful in the past?

Most pathologists are trained to use dead, stained tissues and light field microscopes. Using dark field microscopes and living cells is a more effective way to observe and identify bacteria and fungus in tissue and blood samples.

"An investment in knowledge pays the best interest."

-Benjamin Franklin

"For about 100 years, the scientific community repeatedly changed its collective mind over what viruses are. First seen as poisons, then as life forms, then biological chemicals." -Dr. Luis Villarreal, virologist

SUMMARY

1. Viruses are poisons.
2. Viruses are not cells. They cannot replicate.
3. Viruses are not identified like bacteria and fungus. Most are never identified.
4. HIV is not AIDS. Some HIV drugs can cause AIDS and kill patients.
5. Many viral disease symptoms are caused by fungus and the viruses they excrete.
6. Viruses excreted by fungus contain DNA.
7. Antibiotics cannot kill viruses, because viruses are not living cells.
8. Natural and man-made viruses can infect and kill cells.
9. Antibiotics are viruses.

*Vaccines are
biological and
chemical weapons.*

CHAPTER FIVE

Vaccine Secrets

*"The greatest threat of childhood diseases lies in
the dangerous and ineffectual efforts made
to prevent them through mass immunizations."
-Dr. Robert S. Mendelsohn, Pediatrician*

Vaccines are used to introduce pathogens and poisons into our bodies. The purpose of infecting people with germs and poisons is to create immunity. The word immune means protected against or exempt from something.

Vaccines don't protect us from future infections. We don't become immune to germs and viruses after we are exposed to them. Our bodies must constantly control and neutralize them.

*"The immune system is a network of cells,
tissues, and organs that work together to defend
the body against attacks by foreign invaders."
-Department of Health and Human Services*

Drug companies have been causing infections and death using inoculations for many years. Vaccines are a huge money maker for some drug companies. Selling vaccines are the "bread and butter" of many veterinarians and pediatricians.

45

Mandatory rabies shots for cats and dogs are a good example of how pet owners are forced to infect their pets with pathogens and poisons. Why would a pet need rabies booster shots if they created permanent immunity?

TETANUS VACCINE

"Because a tetanus infection doesn't make the body immune to subsequent infections...the full series of vaccinations must be given after the person recovers."
-Merck Manual

The *Merck Manual* specifically states a tetanus (bacteria) infection doesn't make the body immune to subsequent infections. If that's true, then how can becoming infected over and over by tetanus shots create immunity?

The truth is, it can't. Acquired immunity is a myth that has been promoted by vaccine makers.

ANTIBODIES AND WHITE BLOOD CELLS

"Antibody; a protein produced in the body to neutralize a toxin or other antigen." -Webster's New World Dictionary

White blood cells help kill germs and neutralize poisons. If you become deficient in white blood cells, your body can't control fungus, bacteria and parasites.

"Fungi are everywhere. There are approximately 1.5 million species of fungi on earth, but only about 300 of those are known to make people sick." -CDC

It's a myth that white blood cells create a new type of antibody protein to kill each type of germ. White blood cells don't have tiny laboratories where they go to create antibodies. They use the same proteins to kill all species of bacteria and fungus.

It's also a myth that white blood cells can remember specific germs. White blood cells have a short lifespan of a few days. How can dead cells remember?

"Prior research has indicated that white blood cells produce hydrogen peroxide to kill bacteria."
-Harvard Medical School

When white blood cells release hydrogen peroxide to kill pathogens and neutralize viruses, the release is called a respiratory burst. Hydrogen and oxygen cause molecular damage to the other microbes and alter the viruses.

It's also a myth that antibody proteins can remember specific germs. Antibody proteins are chemicals, not living cells.

Hydrogen peroxide and enzymes are found in a healthy bloodstream. White blood cells also release hydrogen peroxide and other proteins to neutralize viruses and destroy harmful organisms.

47

Hydrogen peroxide is found in raw whole foods and is created by your body. Raw foods provide hydrogen peroxide, bicarbonate, enzymes and vitamin C which help us tolerate and eliminate germs and poisons.

Immunoglobulin is another word for antibody. IgA, IgG, IgD, IgE and IgM are five types of immunoglobulins. These proteins are not created after being exposed to germs and viruses. **They are natural proteins found in a healthy body.**

SEXUALLY TRANSMITTED DISEASES

Syphilis is a disease caused by bacteria and the viruses it excretes. They cause pox and other symptoms. No one becomes immune to syphilis after they get it once.

Prostitutes and promiscuous people don't become immune to sexually transmitted bacteria, fungus, parasites and the viruses they excrete. Their bodies must kill and neutralize them each time.

The continual use of antibiotics and other drugs can cause AIDS and eventually death.

MUTATING VIRUSES

Why don't people become immune to the flu virus if they get it every year? Part of the acquired immunity mythology is the mutating viruses. If scientists can't see viruses using microscopes, how do they know they are mutating? There is no possible way. Viruses are non-living poisons.

TOLERANCE TO POISON

Every time your body is infected by a pathogen or poison, you must be strong enough to tolerate it until your body can eliminate it. Some people can tolerate and eliminate more pathogens and poisons than others. Newborn babies and elderly people are the weakest and most vulnerable.

Human beings can develop some tolerance to poisons, but not immunity to them. Poisons like snake venom, alcohol, antibiotics and man-made chemicals in processed foods cause cell damage regardless of the tolerance factor. Pathogens and viruses can overwhelm the body and cause AIDS, not immunity.

Poisons kill millions of people every year in the world. They cause death if the dose is too large for the body and white blood cells to neutralize. People who have a low tolerance to poisons become ill easier. Some people die from a bee sting or fungus viruses on peanuts.

NATURAL IMMUNITY

It's a myth that a baby develops its immune system by being breast fed. Healthy unborn babies make their own white blood cells and antibody proteins. They are also exposed to mom's antibody proteins before birth.

Mom doesn't have hundreds of different types of antibody proteins. She can't give the baby immunity, but she can make it stronger, so it can tolerate and eliminate more pathogens and poisons. **If a baby doesn't have its own healthy white blood cells and antibody proteins before birth, it will die.**

49

Mothers' milk is the best food for a baby. It contains minerals, fats, antibody proteins, enzymes and many other essential nutrients. Colostrum is a form of milk which has the highest concentration of these nutrients.

Processed baby formulas and pasteurized cow's milk are unnatural foods. They both can cause allergic reactions. Some raw dairy products can be healthy, if the animals are healthy and fed the proper diet.

HEREDITY PROBLEMS

Some babies are born infected with harmful bacteria, fungus or other parasites. The unborn baby can be exposed to whatever is in the mother's body, because the mother and baby share the same blood. Unborn babies receive vitamins, minerals, oxygen and other nutrients from their mothers.

The healthier mom is, the healthier the baby can be at birth. Many babies are born with birth defects because of mineral deficiencies, infections or poisons.

BIOCHEMICAL WEAPONS

"If we do a really great job on new vaccines, healthcare and reproductive healthcare services, we could lower the population by 10 to 15 percent." - Bill Gates

As pediatricians have increased the number of vaccines and antibiotics given to children, the number of children who develop autism disorders, cancer, thrombosis, diabetes and other fungal diseases have also increased.

In 2015 the CDC recommended 49 shots by the age of six and 69 shots by the age of 18. The same shots are given over and over. The hepatitis B vaccine is given seven times by age two. If vaccines actually create immunity, why are children given seven shots?

Why does the herpes virus keep coming back over and over if exposure to a virus causes permanent immunity?

Doctors believe chicken pox and shingles symptoms are created by the same herpes virus. When you are a child the symptoms are called chicken pox and when you get the same symptoms again as an adult, doctors call it shingles. Isn't this more evidence we don't acquire immunity to pathogens and viruses?

"Cancer was practically unknown until compulsory vaccination with cowpox vaccine began to be introduced. I have never seen a case of cancer in an unvaccinated person." -Dr. W. B. Clarke

UNVACCINATED MYTH

Have you ever wondered how an unvaccinated child can infect a fully vaccinated child? How can a vaccinated person become infected if the shots actually work?

Pediatricians may blame the unvaccinated child, or the vaccinated child's weak immune system. They rarely blame the shots, which don't create immunity.

FLU VACCINATION

"In 1918 and 1919 while fighting the flu in the U.S. public health service, it was brought to my attention that rarely anyone who had been thoroughly alkalizing with bicarbonate of soda contracted the disease." -Dr. Volney S. Cheney

An elderly neighbor of mine named Bailey got a flu shot one year. He ended up in the hospital and almost died. Bailey warned me to never get a flu shot. Flu shots have been linked to many diseases, including cancer and dementia. Many doctors and nurses avoid vaccinations.

POLIO DECEPTION

"The injection of any serum, vaccine, or even penicillin has shown a very marked increase in the incidence of polio, at least by 400%." -Dr. William Koch

It is a myth that polio was eliminated by vaccinations. Polio is a word used to classify symptoms such as muscular paralysis. The conventional medical industry is deceiving the public by calling polio symptoms Aseptic Meningitis, Guillian-Barre, Rheumatic fever, Rye's syndrome, Bell's Palsy and Infantile Paralysis. The name has been changed from polio, but the symptoms are still the same. Polio symptoms are often caused by fungus and the viruses they excrete.

"Bell's Palsy is a paralysis or weakness of the muscles on one side of the face. Most cases are thought to be caused by the herpes virus." -Web MD

FEEDLOT POLIO AND MAD COW DISEASE

"There are four main metabolic diseases feedlot operators need to be aware of: polio, acidosis, rumentitis and bloat."
-Steven C. Loerch, Ohio State University

Feedlot polio is caused by feeding cattle large quantities of grains which contain fungus, mycotoxins and man-made poisons. The use of poisonous vaccines, antibiotics and steroids also cause disease symptoms. Mad cow disease symptoms are caused by poisons.

Some of the symptoms caused by poisons are convulsions, lack of coordination, blurred vision, lesions, paralysis, tremors, grinding teeth, groaning, foaming of the mouth, insanity, difficulty breathing, coma and death.

SMALLPOX

"The term "smallpox" was first used in Britain in the 15th century to distinguish variola from the "great pox" (syphilis)." -Wikipedia

Smallpox is a disease name given to symptoms caused by viruses. It is a myth smallpox symptoms have been eradicated by the use of vaccines. Smallpox and syphilis are different names for similar symptoms.

"Some outbreaks of cowpox in cows in North America and Europe were due to infection with vaccinia from recently vaccinated persons." -Merck Veterinarian Manual

The *Merck Veterinarian Manual* believes some disease outbreaks are caused by vaccinated people. Vaccines contain pathogens and poisons which can cause disease outbreaks.

AUTISM

"The only safe vaccine is a vaccine that is never used."
¬James R. Shannon, National Institute of Health

Autism is a brain disorder which mystifies most doctors and scientists and was originally called childhood schizophrenia. Autism is a mental condition, characterized by difficulty in communicating, aggressiveness, self-injury, seizures, repetitive behaviors, etc. Many experts believe the brain damage occurs before the age of three.

Autism Spectrum Disorder (ASD) is used to classify the many symptoms of a malfunctioning brain. ASD symptoms are given names, such as Asperger's syndrome, dyslexia, bipolar, schizophrenia, ADD and ADHD.

ASD symptoms can be caused by antibiotics, fungus, aluminum, mercury, and many other harmful substances in vaccines.

Chemicals in the air, processed foods and water also contribute to autism spectrum disorders. Refined sugars, grains and caffeine can cause brain chemistry disorders and blood sugar diseases such as diabetes and hypoglycemia.

"No batch of vaccine can be proven safe before it is given to children." - Leonard Schule, U.S. Surgeon General

"A UC Davis study found that before 1990, nine in 10,000 kids were diagnosed with autism by age six."
-Lyanne Melendez, ABC News

"About 1 in 68 children has been identified with autism spectrum disorder. About 1 in 6 children in the U.S. had a developmental disability in 2006-2008."
-Center for Disease Control and Prevention

In 2015, approximately 1 in every 50 children, develop autistic symptoms. By the year 2020, 1 in every 5 children may have autistic symptoms because of more pathogens and poisons entering their bodies.

Many children with severe autistic symptoms received large amounts of antibiotics and/or many shots at one time, which overwhelmed their bodies.

Antibiotics and vaccines poison beneficial bacteria and cause microbial imbalances. Beneficial bacteria is needed to digest food, create hormones and neurotransmitters for proper brain function.

Many children with autistic symptoms have become well by changing their diet and cleansing their brains of fungus, heavy metals and toxins. They also gave their bodies the nutrients and beneficial bacteria required to operate properly. The brain chemistry and intestinal flora must be restored to normal.

Millions of children in the U.S. are drugged everyday. They are given psychotropic drugs which cause more mental problems. Amphetamines and other drugs don't solve the problem, but they do cause brain damage and drug addiction.

AUTOIMMUNE DISEASES

The definition of autoimmune disease is an illness that occurs when the body tissues are attacked by white blood cells and antibodies. This definition is incorrect.

Most doctors believe autoimmune diseases such as leukemia are caused by mutated or immature white blood cells attacking the body. They also believe the antibodies released by white blood cells are causing inflammation and cell damage.

People with autoimmune symptoms often take drugs for pain or inflammation. Drugs can't solve problems caused by fungus and poisons in their diet.

ALLERGIES

The definition of an allergy is a hypersensitivity to a specific substance or condition. Most allergic reactions are caused by toxic substances. Milk, wheat, corn, and other processed foods often contain toxins or have been genetically altered.

Fungal infections and poisons weaken the immune system and cause chronic allergies in humans and other animals. Dyes, preservatives and other man-made poisons in processed human and pet foods cause allergic reactions.

Hay fever symptoms can be caused by spores, as well as poisonous pollen and other foreign substances in the air. Polio outbreaks usually occurred in the summer months when the environment was right for fungus spores to germinate.

Antibiotics and alcohol cause allergic reactions. They kill thousands of people every year because they are poisons. Thousands of Americans accidentally overdose each year from over the counter pain killers and prescription drugs. Side effects are allergic reactions. They are the normal way the body reacts to poisons.

YOUR BODY...YOUR CHOICE

You should decide what goes into your body. Please read the insert that comes with each shot. Learn what's in it and then make an informed decision.

There are no safe or effective vaccines and acquired immunity is a myth. For more information go to **vactruth.com** or **nvic.org.**

"In 2011, the Supreme Court said, vaccines are <u>*unavoidably unsafe*</u>*, there shall be no more product liability for any reason, to a vaccine maker."*

-Barbara Loe Fisher,
National Vaccine Information Center

"There is no convincing scientific evidence that mass inoculations can be credited with eliminating any childhood disease." -Dr. Robert Mendelsohn

SUMMARY

1. Vaccines are biological and chemical weapons. They can cause illness and death in human beings and other animals.
2. Acquired immunity is a myth.
3. White blood cells don't create a different antibody protein for each species of fungus or bacteria.
4. White blood cells have a short lifespan of only a few days.
5. Antibodies are hydrogen peroxide and other natural proteins.
6. Babies don't acquire immunity to germs by their mother's milk or exposure to germs.
7. Autism symptoms have many causes including vaccines and antibiotics. Many autistic children have become healthy again by cleansing their bodies and changing their diet.
8. It's a myth that white blood cells and antibodies cause autoimmune diseases.
9. Allergic reactions are usually caused by poisons.

CHAPTER SIX

Antibiotics And Super Bugs

*"Antibiotic use is associated with an increased risk
of breast cancer."* *-National Cancer Institute*

Antibiotics cause fungal infections, while poisoning human
cells and beneficial bacteria. It's a myth that antibiotics are
selective poisons which only kill harmful bacteria cells. The
word antibiotic means anti-life.

The use of antibiotics save lives, but they can also create a
vicious cycle of fungal infections in human beings and other
animals.

Approximately 50% of the antibiotics produced are given
to animals. Most meat and dairy products, are poisoned with
antibiotics.

STREP THROAT

The streptococcus bacteria normally lives in the mouth and
throat. When doctors take strep throat cultures they should
find streptococcus bacteria in the specimens.

Many sore throats are caused by the accumulation of
poisons and fungal infections. They cause the lymph nodes
and tonsils to become inflamed and painful.

When I was five years old, I suffered from many sore throats and swollen lymph nodes. I sometimes had white patches and lesions on my tongue and tonsils. Each time I went to the doctor, I was diagnosed with strep throat and given a penicillin shot.

The doctor routinely looked at my throat and felt my lymph nodes. He would sometimes take a throat culture, but never waited to see if the cause of my sore throat was fungus.

Eventually a surgeon removed my tonsils. The tonsillectomy didn't solve my health problems. A few months later I developed a high fever and went back into the hospital.

My doctor said I had rheumatic fever. I developed polio symptoms and was partially paralyzed for months. Antibiotics didn't solve my health problems.

SUPER BUGS

Staphylococcus aureus bacteria normally lives in and on our bodies without causing illness. It's classified as a super bug because some strains of staph have a tolerance to several types of antibiotics (methicillin). Some types of staph bacteria have been genetically modified by scientists.

Staphylococcus infections can become life threatening when a person has a deficiency of healthy white blood cells or is exposed to a large amount of the bacteria.

Many people have AIDS before entering the hospital. They become weaker while in the hospital because of germs, surgery, antibiotics, chemotherapy or other treatments.

If some staph bacteria is super dangerous, why haven't most of the doctors, nurses, and other hospital workers died? The staph bacteria isn't super strong. Some patients' immune systems are super weak.

Sometimes doctors harm and even kill their patients by trying one antibiotic after another. They believe the infection is bacterial, when it's actually fungal.

There are germs everywhere. Stethoscopes are rarely sanitized, so they spread bacteria and fungus between patients. Blowing out candles on birthday cakes also spreads germs.

The solution is to build a stronger immune system, not take more antibiotics. Antibiotics can weaken the immune system and cause fungal infections.

BLOOD TRANSFUSIONS

"Blood transfusions can transmit infections caused by bacteria, viruses, and parasites."
-American Cancer Society

Blood transfusions are the cause of many fungal and bacterial infections contracted while in the hospital. Pneumonia, cancer, meningitis and blood poisoning can be caused by microbes and poisons in the transfused blood. **Blood transfusions can cause AIDS by poisoning white blood cells.**

Human blood is typed by the presence or absence of specific antigens in the blood. Antigens are any substances to which the body reacts by releasing antibodies.

61

Some of the symptoms caused by blood transfusions include fever, hives, shortness of breath, pain, fast heart rate, chills, low blood pressure, heart attacks, strokes and death. Doctors call these symptoms allergic reactions. Blood transfusions increase the patient's risk of death because the blood isn't purified by the Red Cross and other blood banks.

"A wide variety of organisms, including bacteria, viruses, prions, and parasites can be transmitted through blood transfusions." -Center for Disease Control and Prevention

Transfused blood can also contain fungus and the viruses they excrete. The fungi colonizes into cancer tumors, white clots, plaques, and other fungal growths.

MYCOBACTERIUM

"The Greek prefix myco- means "fungus" alluding to the way mycobacteria have been observed to grow in a mold-like fashion."-Wikipedia

In 1873 Dr. Gerhard Hansen, discovered the microbe that causes leprosy. He was unable to identify the unknown microbe, so he called the germ mycobacteria.

The problem with the word mycobacteria is that fungus and bacteria are two different types of cells. Hansen said mycobacteria would grow in a mold-like fashion. Mold is a type of fungus.

Leprosy and tuberculosis are caused by mycobacteria. TB kills approximately 2 million men, women and children each year worldwide. Most people with TB and leprosy suffer from malnutrition and fungal infections caused by poor diet. Fungus can infect the lungs and other parts of the body. Tuberculosis and leprosy are great examples of how fungus creates ulcers and tumors. The growth of mycobacteria can cause the loss of circulation and gangrene.

Using antibiotics to kill mycobacteria is a mistake. The conventional treatment for leprosy is made up of three types of antibiotics which routinely kill patients. Antibiotics are given in large doses for months or until the patient dies.

People with leprosy can live for years if they don't receive antibiotic treatment. Antibiotics make people with fungal infections more unhealthy.

Most leprosy patients die from AIDS related complications such as cancer, and pneumonia. Organ failure is also common. Antibiotic poisoning and fungal infections aren't listed as their cause of death.

MYCOPLASMA

The word mycoplasma literally means fungus formed. In 1889 Albert Bernhard Frank, mycologist, thought mycoplasma was a fungus due to the fungus-like characteristics. Mycoplasmas were considered viruses for years, because they are not cells. Mycoplasmas are fungus toxins.

STREPTOMYCES

Streptomyces has been misidentified as a bacteria. The antibiotic called streptomycin is created by using streptomyces. The word myces means fungus and the word mycin means a compound derived from fungus. Streptomyces grows in a fungus-like manner and creates mycelium. Mycelium is the body of fungi.

GENETICALLY MODIFIED BACTERIA

"Genetically modified bacteria were the first organisms to be modified in the laboratory, due to their simple genetics."
-Wikipedia, Genetically modified bacteria

Bacteria is being modified by scientists, not mutating because of antibiotics. Some species of bacteria have a tolerance to antibiotics, but not immunity to them.

SUMMARY

1. Antibiotics save lives, but they also cause fungal infections.
2. Antibiotics kill human and beneficial bacteria cells.
3. Mycobacteria is a type of fungus and mycoplasmas are fungi viruses.
4. Some species of fungus are misidentified as bacteria.
5. Fungus and bacteria have been genetically modified by scientists.
6. Antibiotic use is associated with an increased risk of breast cancer.

SECTION TWO

How To
Create A Healthy Body

*"We must become
a nation of prevention.
We were too long
a nation of treatment."*

*-Richard Carmona,
U.S. Surgeon General*

*"Death by
refined sugar
may not be an
overstatement."*

-Dr. Joseph Mercola

CHAPTER SEVEN

Symptom Solutions

"I'm a realist, as long as the profit is in the treatment of symptoms, rather than the search for causes, that's where the medical profession will go for its harvest."
-Arthur F. Coca, M.D.

A disease is a particular destructive process or imbalance in an organism. When a body is malfunctioning, it creates symptoms. Doctors are trained to examine patients and then give their symptoms disease names.

Conventional doctors often treat symptoms with poisonous drugs, without knowing the cause of the destructive process or imbalance.

Toxicity, malnutrition, constipation, dehydration, fungal infections, and too much tension all contribute to a poorly functioning body. Whatever you eat, breathe, drink and think, affects how your body functions.

ACID-ALKALINE BALANCE

The body is continually trying to maintain order or balance. The brain regulates body temperature, blood sugar and many other functions. Poisons cause a pH imbalance in the body.

They cause molecular, hormonal, mineral and microbial imbalances. Poisons create a low oxygen bloodstream, inflammation and pain in the body. There are good and bad acids. Essential fatty acids in meats and acids found in apples and other foods are good for you. The bad acids are poisons. These bad acids are usually man-made chemicals or toxins excreted by plants, animals or microorganisms.

Sucrose, processed grains and alcohol are just three substances which poison the body, and create an acidic, low oxygen bloodstream. This condition is called toxemia or acidosis.

"The sugar of commerce is nothing but crystallized acid."
-Dr. Robert Bolsler

ACIDOSIS

"Acidosis is the most important nutritional problem that feedlots face daily and is a major challenge for dairies as well." - Dr. Clell V. Bagley D.V.M.

Acidosis is a condition in which there is an abnormal retention of acid or loss of alkali in the body. Grain overload, also called acidosis, causes disease and death in livestock. Bovine Respiratory Disease symptoms are caused by stress, vaccines, fungus, antibiotics and poisoned grains.

Some of the symptoms of poisoning in cattle are vitamin deficiency, poor immune function, infections, founder, lameness, ulcers, bloating, diarrhea, sudden death syndrome, kidney failure, shock and death.

Cattle are grass eaters. When they are fed poisonous grains it creates an acidic, low oxygen environment. All of the poisons kill beneficial bacteria and white blood cells, which help control fungus. The cattle can then develop systemic fungal infections.

When human beings eat processed grains and refined sugars, it causes fungus to ferment and excrete viruses. As people consume more processed foods which are poisoned, they develop digestive problems such as irritable bowel syndrome, celiac disease, acid reflux disease and leaky gut syndrome. Acid reflux disease is chronic acid indigestion.

FUNGUS ACIDS

The powerful mind-altering drug called LSD is made from ergot fungus. Another name for LSD is acid. Ergot toxins cause symptoms such as spasms, diarrhea, anxiety, hallucinations, stupor, mania, psychosis, headaches, nausea and vomiting, ulcers, pain, blisters, loss of circulation, gangrene, rash and burning feelings.

Fungi has been killing human beings for thousands of years. Many disease epidemics in the past and present are caused by fungi and the viruses they excrete.

ACIDS AND CALCIFICATION

"Fungus can cause elevated blood calcium by the alcohol they excrete. Calcium is an essential nutrient for healthy bones, and alcohol is its enemy." -Web MD

69

Alcohol is a poison excreted by fungus. The body uses calcium to neutralize poisons, which increases the level of calcium in the bloodstream. Calcium and fungus can bind to form plaque on the teeth, arteries, joints, brain, liver, pancreas, or anywhere in the body.

This destructive process also causes stones, bone spurs, loss of circulation, arthritis and other autoimmune disorders. Diabetics lose circulation in their legs and feet because of fungus and calcium build up in blood vessels. The body leeches calcium from bones to neutralize acids, causing osteoporosis.

"Refined sugar upsets the calcium-phosphorus ratio in the blood more than any other single factor." -Dr. Melvin Page

Antacids and calcium supplements help cause calcification of the body if the calcium isn't absorbed into the bones or flushed out of the body. As toxins, calcium and fungi accumulate in organs and tissues, the body malfunctions.

AUTO-BREWERY SYNDROME

In a brewery, the oxygen and sugar levels are controlled inside each vat to produce the desired amount of alcohol. As the oxygen is reduced the yeast will excrete more alcohol.

Auto-Brewery Syndrome is a medical condition in which the fungus living in your body creates alcohol. Refined sugars and processed grains poison blood cells, while feeding the yeast. The alcohol excreted by the fungus also poisons the body causing cell damage, inflammation and calcification.

When there is plenty of oxygen in the bloodstream, anaerobic fungus cells don't create as much alcohol. They mainly excrete carbon dioxide like human cells.

Fungus can go anywhere in the body, including the bones and brain, when there are not enough white blood cells to stop them. As the fungus colonizes it creates growths that doctors call tumors, scarring, sclerosis, plaques, white clots, etc.

HEART DISEASE AND FUNGUS

"About 12.9 million people worldwide died from some form of cardiovascular disease in 2004."
-World Health Organization

Heart disease is the number one killer of Americans. Over 600,000 men, women and children die every year from heart disease.

Dr. Robert C. Atkins proved it was a myth that animal cholesterol causes heart disease. In his book, *Dr. Atkins' New Diet Revolution,* he described how refined carbohydrates are causing heart disease.

"Cardiovascular disease is the biggest killer of apes in captivity." -*USA TODAY*

Cleveland Metroparks Zoo changed the diet of their western lowland gorillas, because they were dying from heart disease. The gorillas were overweight and suffering from many chronic diseases.

They were not eating animal products.

71

Zookeepers were feeding their gorillas monkey biscuits. Their diet consisted of 25-50% processed biscuits which were similar to human cookies. They contained refined sugars, grains and other harmful ingredients which poisoned the gorillas. The refined sugar and flour caused calcium build up and fungal growths. They also caused blood sugar imbalances, acidosis and obesity.

"Primates can be fed a diet based on commercial monkey biscuits or canned primate or marmoset diet."
-Merck Veterinarian Manual

The Merck Veterinarian Manual was wrong. The gorillas became healthy when they stopped eating the processed biscuits. Gorillas at the Cleveland Metroparks Zoo now eat a natural raw food diet like gorillas in the wild.

"The Cleveland Metroparks Zoo stopped feeding the male western lowland gorillas processed biscuits and they are much healthier now."
-Dr. Pam Dennis, Cleveland Metroparks Zoo

CHILDHOOD HEART DISEASE

"Inflammation is involved in all stages of arteriosclerosis."
-Harvard Medical School

Many children die every year from heart disease. Even newborn babies can die from heart attacks and strokes. When children die from heart attacks and strokes the doctors call the disease childhood thrombosis.

How is that possible if heart disease is caused by the build up of animal cholesterol? Many babies are born already infected with fungus. Their plaques and white clots are fungal growths. **Fungus and human cells are eukaryotic cells, which contain cholesterol and DNA.**

"Inflammation appears connected to almost every known chronic disease." -Dr. Mark Hyman

Inflammation is redness, pain, heat, and swelling in the body, due to poisons, injury, infections, etc. When cells are damaged by an injury or poisons, inflammation is created.

WHITE CLOTS

"We need to understand why people who get transfusions are more likely to get blood clots." -Charles Francis, M.D.

The definition of the word clot is a soft clump or a thickened mass. There are two types of clots. Red blood clots are caused by red blood platelets, usually when a person is injured. White clots are fungal growths.

Cardiologists and pathologists don't know what white clots really are and why they are formed. Suzanne Somers proved cancer tumors and white clots are colonizing fungi. Blood is one way of transmitting antigens, such as fungus.

Cardiologists call a white clot thrombus. A piece of thrombus floating in the blood is called an embolus.

Thromboembolism is a leading cause of illness and death in cancer patients. The use of birth control pills and cancer treatments cause white blood clots to form. Rheumatic heart disease is a good example of how heart disease is caused by fungal infections.

PLAQUE

Atherosclerosis is a disease characterized by the formation of plaques. Arteriosclerosis is the thickening and hardening of the walls of the arteries.

Arterial plaques are raised patches that don't cover the entire artery. If plaques did, then bypass surgery would be impossible. The whole artery would need to be replaced.

The American Heart Association doesn't know what causes atherosclerosis. The popular **theory or guess** is that plaque buildup is caused by animal cholesterol.

*"Exactly how atherosclerosis begins or what causes
it isn't known, but some theories have been proposed."*
-American Heart Association

Plaque can be bio-film, raised patches or lesions. Some plaques contain a soft cheese-like substance. Yeast infections in other parts of the body can create similar cheese-like substances.

Patches can be found on the walls of arteries or brain tissues in Alzheimer's and Parkinson's patients. Plaques can grow anywhere in or on the body. They can sometimes be found in the body by doing a coronary calcium scan or using ultra-sound equipment.

Aspirin can reduce the risk of heart disease because it reduces fungal growths and thins the blood. Aspirin is an unhealthy way to prevent heart disease. People having a heart attack are often given aspirin to thin the blood and reduce pain.

"Plaque, a sticky film of bacteria, constantly forms on your teeth. When you eat or drink foods containing sugars, the bacteria produce acids that attack tooth enamel."
-American Dental Association

Dentists have been taught dental plaque is made of bacteria cells. They know very little about fungus and the formation of plaque.

Plaque on teeth is caused by minerals, bacteria and fungus cells hardening on the teeth. Cavities are mainly caused by refined sugars and chemicals, which dissolve tooth enamel. Facultative bacteria and fungus don't excrete harmful acids unless they are fermenting. Refined sugars cause fermenting.

"There are a lot of studies that suggest that oral health, and gum disease in particular are related to serious conditions like heart disease."
-Sally Cram, D.D.S., American Dental Association

There is a connection between plaque on teeth and the walls of arteries. Fibrosis, psoriasis, cirrhosis, and sclerosis are different words used for plaque buildup. They involve thickening and hardening of tissues caused by calcium and fungus cells.

PSORIASIS

The skin condition called psoriasis is a good example of plaque buildup. Over seven million Americans suffer from psoriasis, and 80% of those people have plaque psoriasis. Eighty million men, women and children are affected worldwide by this type of fungal infection.

Psoriasis is considered an autoimmune disease. Plaque psoriasis can occur in the brain, pancreas, liver, kidneys, joints, arteries, veins or anywhere in the body. Psoriasis causes inflammation, lesions, and white patches. As the fungus growths become larger, they cause the liver, brain, pancreas and other parts of the body to malfunction.

"Psoriasis can occur on any part of the body and is associated with other serious health conditions, such as diabetes, heart diseases and depression."
-National Psoriasis Foundation

There is a connection between psoriasis and many other chronic diseases. That connection is fungal infections.

SYSTEMIC SCLEROSIS

"Systemic sclerosis causes an overproduction of collagen and other proteins in various tissues. The cause is unknown. Systemic sclerosis often causes damage that is widespread throughout the body. No treatment changes the course of this disorder." -Merck Manual

Sclerosis isn't causing over-production of collagen and other proteins. Sclerosis is the buildup of scar tissue, fungus and calcium. The definition of the word sclerosis is an abnormal hardening of body tissues. Multiple sclerosis and ALS are caused by fungus.

CHOLESTEROL

Green vegetables contain the same waxy substance most doctors have been taught causes heart attacks and strokes. All healthy human cells contain the hormone called cholesterol. Cholesterol is found in healthy plant, animal and fungus cells.

"There is a widespread belief among the public and even among chemists that plants don't contain cholesterol."
-E.J. Behrman, M.D.

Some fats are healthy while others are unhealthy. Processed vegetable oils cause inflammation as they damage cells. Vegetable oils are unnatural and have been created by using poisonous chemicals. The poisons and altered molecules cause inflammation as they destroy healthy cells.

"Grass fed animals rich in all the fats, are now proven to be health enhancing." -Dr. Joseph Mercola

ESKIMOS

"Old age sets in at fifty and its signs are strongly marked at sixty." - Dr. Samuel Hutton, Studied the Eskimos 1902-1913

Heart disease is not caused by animal cholesterol. Eskimos of the far north lived almost exclusively on a diet of fish, seals and other animals. They ate large amounts of raw animal fat, but they didn't die from cancer or heart disease at a young age. The raw foods provided large amounts of C and B vitamins. The Eskimos were much healthier before they started eating processed foods.

Present day Inuit Indians who eat a lot of poisoned foods and drink coffee, sodas, and alcohol suffer from chronic degenerative diseases. They are dying from cancer, diabetes, asthma, heart attacks and strokes. Processed foods cause nutritional deficiencies and fungal infections.

STATINS AND DEMENTIA

Statins are one of the world's bestselling drugs. Cholesterol screening is used to scare people into taking statins. The theory of high and low cholesterol is used to sell statin drugs.

Statins are suppose to lower cholesterol in the body. They are poisons made of synthetic chemicals or fungus toxins.

Every cell in the body needs cholesterol to function properly. Statins have been linked to dementia, because they cause a lack of cholesterol in brain cells.

Calcification, dehydration, fungus, heavy metal and chemical poisoning can also cause the brain to malfunction. Cleansing the brain and proper diet are essential if you want to become healthy.

PARKINSON'S SYNDROME

*"We have **no solid theory** of what causes Parkinson's disease. The drugs available now are designed to help reduce symptoms but **don't attack their cause.**"*
-James Beck, Parkinson's Disease Foundation

The actor Michael J. Fox suffers from a chronic disease called Parkinson's Disease. When Michael was living in the country of Bhutan, his Parkinson's symptoms vanished. When he returned to the United States, so did his symptoms. What could cause his temporary cure?

First, he stopped eating his usual diet and ate like the natives. He stopped poisoning himself with processed American food.

Second, he was living at a high altitude which contributed to his bloodstream becoming more alkaline. Alkalosis can be caused by rapid, deep breathing or being at high altitude. The pancreas releases more bicarbonate into the bloodstream which helps alter the pH level of the blood.

Michael's pancreas probably neutralized the fungus toxins by releasing more bicarbonate. Pancreatic juice is composed of digestive enzymes and bicarbonate.

Plaques and Lewy bodies are fungal growths. The brain damage created by fungus and the powerful viruses they excrete cause Parkinson's symptoms.

Most chronic degenerative diseases are caused by poisons, pathogens and degenerated foods.

ARTHRITIS

There are two types of arthritis: osteoarthritis and rheumatoid arthritis. Rheumatoid arthritis is a chronic disease with painful swelling of joints which often leads to deformity.

.

79

Arthritis is classified as an autoimmune disease. People who have psoriatic arthritis usually have skin psoriasis.

Both types of arthritis are caused mainly by processed foods. Refined vegetable oils, sugars and grains cause inflammation, calcium imbalance and fungal infections. The body cannot function properly while being poisoned.

Gout can be caused by alcohol you drink, or alcohol excreted by fungus growing in your body. Gout is not caused by eating healthy meats. Eskimos ate large amounts of meats and didn't suffer from gout. Human beings have been consuming alcoholic beverages and refined sugar for hundreds of years and suffering the consequences of it. Fungus thrive on refined sugars and grains.

Bone spurs, loss of cartilage and bone density, pain and inflammation are part of the process. Rheumatoid arthritis is caused by fungus plaque and mineral crystals in the bones and joints. The fungus destroys tissues as it grows and excretes alcohol.

Bone on bone in joints can be caused by calcium deposits, not lack of cartilage. Bone spurs are a good example of this phenomenon.

Osteoporosis is a bone disorder marked by porous, brittle bones. The body leeches calcium from the bones to neutralize alcohol and other harmful poisons. The alcohol excreted by fungus kills cells, causing pain and inflammation.

Enbrel and Humira are good examples of drugs which poison white blood cells and cause systemic fungal infections. Their television commercials list fungal infections as a side effect when taking these poisonous drugs.

CYSTIC FIBROSIS AND FIBROMYALGIA

Fibrosis is defined as an excessive growth of fibrous connective tissue. Fibroids are defined as benign tumors of muscular and fibrous tissues, typically developing in the wall of the uterus. The same phenomenon is happening when a person has fibromyalgia. Fungus is the fibrous connective tissue.

Cystic fibrosis is a disease marked by fibrosis of the pancreas and by frequent lung infections. A cyst is a sac-like structure in plants or animals, filled with diseased matter.

APLASTIC AND SICKLE CELL ANEMIA

"Most episodes of sickle cell crisis last between five and seven days. Although infection, dehydration, and acidosis can act as triggers, in most instances no predisposing cause is identified." -Wikipedia

Leukemia and many autoimmune diseases are caused by fungus, not immature or mutated white blood cells. Drugs, fungus cells and their toxins cause symptoms such as infection, dehydration and acidosis.

"Causes of aplastic anemia include infections, drugs and autoimmune diseases." -Mayo Clinic

Anemia is a condition marked by a deficiency of healthy red blood cells, resulting in low oxygen and weakness. One cause of anemia is poisons which destroy red blood cells.

81

Sickle cell and aplastic anemia are also caused by fungus and their toxins which affect the bone marrow and stem cells.

HEPATITIS AND CIRRHOSIS

"Cirrhosis is a slowly progressing disease in which healthy liver tissue is replaced with scar tissue."-WebMD

Cirrhosis and hepatitis are caused by poisons and fungal infections in the liver. As the fungus colonizes and excretes alcohol, it damages cells and causes calcium build up. The fungus, scar tissue and calcium cause the liver to slowly harden and malfunction. The good news is, the liver can regenerate itself when you stop poisoning your body.

CATARACTS

Cataracts are the leading cause of blindness in the world. Doctors don't know for sure what causes them. The thick, hardened cloudy tissues in the eye is made up of calcium, toxins and sometimes fungus. During surgery an ultrasound device is used to break up the hard calcified tissues. Doctors also use ultrasound to break up kidney stones.

Chemotherapy, steroids, alcohol and infections have been know to cause cataracts. Poisons, such as sucrose create unstable sugar, oxygen and calcium levels in the blood. According to the American Diabetic Association people with diabetes are 60% more likely to develop cataracts.

KIDNEY DISEASE

Over 48,000 Americans die each year from kidney disease because of processed foods and a lack of enough clean water. Kidney, gallbladder, pancreas and liver stones are caused by blood calcium imbalance and acids. The body is using calcium to neutralize poisons. The stones are similar to bone spurs. The same process causes arthritis. Fungus and calcium deposits can build up inside any organ and then cause it to malfunction.

DIABETES

Over 68,000 Americans per year die of heart disease related to diabetes. Most diabetics die from heart attacks, strokes and kidney failure caused by fungus and calcium build up. Refined foods cause fungus and calcium build up in the pancreas and other organs which causes them to malfunction. Eating processed foods, especially refined sugars, grains and alcoholic beverages cause blood sugar imbalances and acidosis. Refined sugars cause a blood sugar roller coaster ride.

Most doctors and the American Diabetes Association still believe refined sugar doesn't cause diabetes. Some doctors tell their patients to eat candy if they have low blood sugar and then use insulin if it becomes too high. The refined sugar roller coaster is a dangerous ride.

The blood sugar balance is vital to proper functioning of the body. Diabetic people lose blood circulation because of fungus growths and calcium deposits in blood vessels. The loss of circulation leads to blindness, amputations and eventually heart attacks and strokes.

83

Low sugar and oxygen in the bloodstream can cause mental problems, such as depression, bipolar disorder and schizophrenia symptoms. Chronic blood sugar imbalances are called diabetes and hypoglycemia.

Refined sugar is similar to the drug methamphetamine in many ways. They are both poisons which destroy tooth enamel and cause imbalances in the body. They both suppress the immune system and cause fungal infections.

Unhealthy foods cannot produce healthy bodies.

LUNG DISEASES

Lung diseases are one of the leading causes of death in the U.S. Over 137,000 Americans die from lung diseases every year. Lung diseases can be caused by many different things including bacteria, fungus and foreign materials in the lungs. Emphysema is not lung cancer.

LUNG CANCER

"Every year, about 16,000 to 24,000 Americans die of lung cancer, even though they have never smoked." -ACS

Harmful chemicals in tobacco poison red and white blood cells. When the body becomes deficient in white blood cells, the facultative fungus then thrive. They colonize in the lungs and create cancer tumors.

ASTHMA, TB, COLDS AND FLU

Many people with asthma, tuberculosis and other fungal infections move to low humidity areas like Arizona. Fungus doesn't grow as well in a low moisture environment. Winter is the flu season in cold weather areas. The lack of fresh air inside homes weakens the immune system and helps mold grow. Cold and flu symptoms are often caused by fungus and the viruses they excrete.

"In the Northern hemisphere, winter is the time for flu."
-Center for Disease Control and Prevention.

HOSPITAL CARE

"A hospital is like a war. You should try your best to stay out of it." -Dr. Robert S. Mendelsohn

A hospital is a dangerous place to stay. They are filled with germs, stale air and the food is usually unhealthy. **Over 400,000 Americans die each year from medical errors and infections they contract while staying in the hospital.**
A good mechanic will use accurate knowledge and logical thinking to diagnose and then repair an automobile. If the vehicle isn't fixed correctly, the mechanic may not get paid. Doctors and hospitals make more money when there are medical complications such as infections and errors.

"Hospitals are a business, after all, and the more services used by any patient the more money they make. Medical errors are good for business." -Dr. Joseph Mercola

85

UNNECESSARY SURGERIES

"Greed plays a role in causing unnecessary surgery. If you eliminated all unnecessary surgery, most surgeons would go out of business." - Robert Mendelsohn, M.D.

Some physical injuries and birth defects require necessary surgery. The CDC says there are approximately 50 million surgeries performed in the U.S. each year. Most are unnecessary or useless.

APPENDECTOMIES

Surgeons perform over 293,000 appendectomies every year in the U.S. at an average cost of $33,000. Appendicitis usually occurs because of hardened stool or gas. Most constipation problems can be solved using laxatives or warm water enemas.

If you go to the emergency room, the odds are good the surgeon will want to operate. Surgeries are a big money maker for hospitals.

CESAREAN SURGERY

Cesarean surgeries (1.4 million in 2007) are very popular and usually unnecessary. There was a time when women squatted or used birthing chairs when having a baby. Women were sometimes helped by midwives.

86

Having women lie on their backs interferes with natural childbirth. Doctors sometimes use drugs to reduce pain or knock out mothers. How can a woman dilate properly when she is drugged? The babies are also being drugged. Obstetricians and hospitals have created new ways to make more money from something as natural as childbirth.

HYSTERECTOMIES AND MASTECTOMIES

Hysterectomies are another big money maker for surgeons. Approximately 600,000 hysterectomies are performed each year in the U.S. Women who suffer from chronic yeast infections are targeted for hysterectomies. The fungi cells colonize and form what doctors call tumors, fibroids, endometriosis, cysts and scar tissue.

Over 200,000 women are diagnosed with breast cancer each year in the U.S. and approximately 100,000 of those women undergo breast removal surgery at an average cost of $35,000. Thousands of fearful women have their healthy breasts removed to prevent breast cancer.

TONSILLECTOMIES

Removing tonsils has been a big money maker for surgeons since the 1950s. Many surgeons believe tonsils are not necessary for good health. Over 1 million tonsillectomies are performed each year in the U.S.

The doctor's solution for chronic sore throats and swollen lymph nodes has been to remove the tonsils. Swollen tonsils and nodes are usually caused by yeast infections, accumulated poisons and mucus in the body.

Surgeons take out thousands of tonsils each year because of snoring or sleep apnea. Removing the tonsils usually doesn't solve the problem.

LIVER TRANSPLANTS

Hepatitis is a Greek and Latin word for a swollen liver. Hepatitis can be caused by alcohol, fungus, prescription drugs, processed foods and other poisons.

When the liver becomes hardened by scarring, calcium and fungus growths, it's called cirrhosis. The liver is an organ that can be cleansed, regenerated and become well again if you stop damaging it. You can cleanse your liver and remove stones using citrus juice, olive oil and clean water.

Liver transplants can cost over $500,000 and some medications can cost as much as $1000 a pill.

GALLBLADDER SURGERY

Approximately 750,000 Americans have gallbladder surgery each year. Many patients suffer bile duct injury during the procedure and die within a year.

The gallbladder can be purged of stones using lemon juice and olive oil. I know people who have successfully removed their gallstones this way.

CURING CHRONIC DISEASES

To cure chronic diseases, we want to identify the cause of the problem, and then focus on the solution. We must sometimes change our beliefs and habits to get well.

GORILLAS AND DISEASE SYMPTOMS

1. The gorillas developed chronic disease symptoms because of processed food and fungal infections.
2. The gorillas were poisoned by the primate biscuits.
3. The gorillas didn't go to rehab, 12 step meetings or see a therapist to cope with their sugar cravings.
4. They didn't go to an alternative or conventional doctor for expensive treatments.
5. They didn't use probiotics, herbs, diet products, juicers, or enema bags.
6. They didn't get acupuncture, massage or chiropractic therapies.
7. They didn't do green juice therapy, water fasting or sauna therapy.
8. They didn't use apple cider vinegar, garlic, olive oil, vitamin C or baking soda.
9. They didn't join a gym, lift weights or vigorously exercise three times every week.
10. They didn't learn yoga or meditation to cope with stress.

They did stop eating poisoned food and gave their bodies the right food to be healthy.

"Good nutrition will prevent 95% of all disease."
-Dr. Linus Pauling, two-time Nobel Prize winner

SUMMARY

1. Processed foods are poisoned foods. They cause metabolic, hormonal, mineral and microbial imbalances. They cause fungal infections.
2. Calcification is caused by poisons.
3. Auto-brewery syndrome is caused by refined sugars, grains and fungus.
4. Cleveland Metroparks Zoo gorillas died from heart disease caused by processed food, not animal cholesterol.
5. Eskimos lived healthy lives, for many years, eating mostly raw animal meats and fats.
6. It's a myth arterial plaque is caused by animal cholesterol.
7. Cholesterol is found in healthy plant, animal and fungus cells.
8. Some babies die from heart disease because of plaque and thrombus growths. The growths are fungus.
9. Statins don't prevent heart disease. They help cause a deficiency of cholesterol and dementia.
10. Most surgeries are unnecessary.
11. Many chronic diseases can be cured by giving your body the nutrients it requires and avoiding poisons.
12. Start taking action to create a healthy body.

*"Whenever a doctor
cannot do good, he must be
kept from doing harm."*

- Hippocrates

"Those who begin to exercise regularly and replace white flour, sugar and devitalized foods with live, organic natural foods begin to feel better immediately."

- Jack Lalanne

CHAPTER EIGHT

Self Healthcare

"The doctor of the future will give no medicine,
but will instruct his patient in the care of the human frame,
in diet and in the cause and prevention of disease."
-Thomas Edison

The definition of the word healthcare is the prevention and treatment of illness or injury on an ongoing basis. The word health means physical and mental well-being. Most disease symptoms are caused by poisons, pathogens and nutritional deficiencies which create imbalances in the body.

The human body is like an automobile which eventually wears out with time and use. There are no pills, plastic surgeries, creams or foods which can keep us young or ageless forever.

The body must be maintained properly or it will break down and wear out faster. Whatever we breathe, eat, drink or think affects our body chemistry. Our bodies are electromagnetic machines which create chemicals and electrical energy.

Whenever stress, poison or poor diet weaken our bodies, we are vulnerable to being killed by microbes. Human beings must cope with poisons, pathogens, tensions, injuries, and our own genetic weaknesses.

93

Our bodies can't function properly on processed foods. People from around the world suffer more diseases when they abandon their primitive organic diets.

Raw whole foods contain more electrical energy, enzymes, and other nutrients than cooked foods. Processed foods lack essential vitamins, minerals, fiber and other nutrients. Most people die from diseases caused by poisons, poor diet and microorganisms.

OKINAWANS

The Japanese people of Okinawa were considered one of the longest living groups of people in the world. At one time, approximately 34 out of 100 Okinawans lived 100 years or more. Okinawans were not vegetarians or vegans.

The Okinawans didn't use poisonous fertilizers and pesticides when growing grains, fruits and vegetables. The water wasn't poisoned with chlorine, fluoride and other man-made chemicals. Their food and water supplied the nutrients they needed without poisoning them. They ate a primitive diet of whole nutrient dense foods grown in mineral rich soil.

Their animals weren't poisoned by toxic grains, vaccines, steroids, antibiotics and genetically modified foods. The animal products they ate didn't cause cancer or heart disease.

The Okinawans were not poisoned by doctors, grocery stores and fast food restaurants. They were not being poisoned by electrical radiation. They were not injected with germs and poisons by annual flu shots and other vaccinations. Okinawans were healthier in the past because of their primitive natural diet and they had less **poisons** in their environment.

GERM THEORY

Claude Bernard said, *"The germ is nothing, the terrain is everything."* The strength of your whole body is vital to combating germs, but germs are far from being nothing. Food and water infected with germs have killed millions of healthy people.

It doesn't matter how healthy you are, if you become infected with germs or the viruses they excrete, you can become seriously ill.

Louis Pasteur is famous for the process called pasteurization. He used heat to kill bacteria cells. Heat can also destroy many of the healthiest nutrients in foods. It appears Pasteur wasn't aware of beneficial bacteria. He may have believed all bacteria was bad.

THE HEALING ART

In the past, the best natural healers used whole organic foods, herbs, water fasting and prayer to help others become well.

Many shamans, witch doctors and medicine men hoarded knowledge. They kept their knowledge secret to gain power and material wealth. They sometimes used their knowledge to control the minds of their followers.

Hippocrates (460-377 B.C.) is considered the father of western medicine. Hippocrates and the healers of his time didn't understand the cause of many disease symptoms. Physicians still don't have all the answers.

95

WHOLE FOOD SHALL BE THY MEDICINE

Our air, water, soil and foods are becoming more poisoned everyday. The water and soil used to grow organic foods are often contaminated. Organically grown foods should have less poisons and more nutrients than processed foods.

Most food in grocery stores, including fruits and vegetables, have been irradiated or poisoned. Irradiation damages the cells and enzymes of food.

Some doctors are aware of how diet affects health. They know we can't live on processed foods and remain healthy. They encourage their patients to eat more natural organic produce. **Raw organic fruits and vegetables are great healers.**

HEALTHCARE BASICS

OXYGEN AND CLEAN AIR

Oxygen is one of the most important nutrients our bodies need. You can go weeks without food and days without water, but only minutes without oxygen. The body requires oxygen and hydrogen to be healthy.

Winter is the cold and flu season in areas with cold weather. A closed up home with stale air suppresses the immune system. Air conditioning can also cause health problems. We need to breathe fresh air.

Our air is being poisoned by automobile and airplane fuel. Some geo-engineering planes are creating toxic chemical trails. These poisons end up in the soil, water and our bodies.

CLEAN WATER

Clean water is vital for good health. Most water is made of oxygen, hydrogen and minerals. Drinking plenty of water is necessary to cleanse out the poisons we accumulate. People can die from dehydration and constipation, because of the build up of toxins.

Human cells must have enough water and minerals to create and conduct electricity. High blood pressure symptoms can be caused by dehydration and thick blood.

If you are suffering from cold or flu symptoms, water will help flush out the fungal and bacterial viruses. Water thins the blood and helps the kidneys filter out poisons. Refined sugars thicken the blood and poisons the body.

The body is made of over 60% water and the brain is over 75% water. Many people with dementia are dehydrated from drinking sodas, tea, coffee or alcohol instead of water. Without enough clean water the brain and pineal gland can become clogged with toxic substances.

City water is often poisoned with chlorine, fluoride and other chemicals. Large amounts of chlorine will kill bacteria cells including the beneficial bacteria in your intestines.

A reverse osmosis filtering system is a good solution for drinking and cleaning food. Filtered, distilled and spring water are healthier choices than city water.

MINERALS

Alkalizing minerals are vital nutrients for maintaining pH balance. We can supply our bodies minerals by water, food and unrefined salt.

97

To be healthy we need whole foods with all of the essential vitamins, enzymes, minerals and other unknown nutrients. Our bodies require foods that haven't been poisoned by chemicals.

Commercial food processing strips away over half of the nutrients. Refined table salt, white flour and table sugar have been stripped of most essential minerals. They have also been bleached and contain other harmful chemicals.

If you choose to use salt, it's best to use unrefined sea or Himalayan salt which contains iodine, selenium and other minerals. Iodine is essential for proper thyroid functioning. Dried kelp is a good source of iodine.

FOOD

Food labeling is a fraud. Boxed, bottled and canned processed foods are poisoned with chemicals. Food manufacturers are not required to be truthful about the ingredients in their foods. Many ingredients are not even listed on the label. The manufacturers also use many names to hide poisonous chemicals such as MSG.

Food pyramids have serious flaws. Eating large amounts of processed grain products causes illness and death. Processed grains in pet foods are unhealthy for dogs and cats too. Primate biscuits made of refined grains cause gorillas to have chronic degenerative diseases.

Refined vegetable oils are unhealthy fats. Harmful chemicals are used to create most vegetable oils. Cold pressed olive, hemp and coconut oils are healthy fats.

Pasteurized and homogenized dairy products can cause health problems, such as lactose intolerance, allergic reactions, mucus, and inflammation. Raw milk is very different from processed milk. They can be alkalizing and healthy. People don't need milk after they are weaned.

Coffee contains a poison called caffeine. It's also a diuretic and causes dehydration. Caffeine causes many side effects and chemical dependency. Many mental and physical disease symptoms, such as blood sugar and brain chemistry imbalances are caused by caffeine.

Wine is unhealthy to drink. The alcohol in wine is poison excreted by yeast. Alcohol causes birth defects, miscarriages, insanity and death. Grapes do contain many healthy nutrients. Eating raw organic grapes is a healthier way to get antioxidants.

Beer and other liquors contain fungus toxins. They intoxicate the whole body and cause the loss of mental and physical control. Alcohol is a powerful mind-altering drug which causes blood sugar and brain chemistry imbalances.

Soda pop is unhealthy to drink. Most soda pop contains refined sweeteners, caffeine, phosphoric acid and other poisonous chemicals. Caffeine and refined sugars are the cause of many mental disorders. They contribute to depression, bipolar disorder, schizophrenia and severe mood swings by causing brain chemistry and blood sugar imbalances.

Energy and sports drinks are unhealthy.

Processed juices often use high pressure processing which damages cells and digestive enzymes. They may also contain harmful chemicals.

Most foods sold at grocery stores are poisoned. Processed foods can contain MSG, bisphenol A, aspartame, bromine and thousands of other poisons.

Genetically modified foods cause disease symptoms. Many kinds of corn and soybeans have been genetically altered and contain harmful bacteria. They poison the body and destroy beneficial bacteria which causes digestive disease symptoms. Some types of alfalfa fed to livestock have been genetically modified and cause disease symptoms in livestock.

Aluminum is inside most baking powders, antiperspirants and antacids. Cooking with aluminum pots can cause poisoning. Many vaccines, such as flu shots, contain aluminum. Aluminum poisoning has been linked to dementia.

Refined sugars cause disease. They contribute to all degenerative diseases. Table sugar, corn syrup and aspartame are harmful sweeteners. Raw honey and unsulfured blackstrap molasses are healthy sweeteners.

Grains are not necessary to maintain a healthy body. Most grains contain pesticides, fungus toxins and other poisons. Commercial breads and other baked goods contain many harmful substances, such as aluminum and bromine. Baker's yeast can cause allergic reactions and disease symptoms. Eating bleached white flour is a leading cause of constipation and digestive disorders. Processed white flour and rice lacks fiber, vitamins, minerals and other nutrients. Some organically grown whole grains can be healthy. Eliminating grains can eliminate many disease symptoms.

Mushrooms are fungal growths and are known to absorb and concentrate poisons from the air, water and soil. According to Dr. Cornelia de Moor, cordycepin derived from mushrooms could have adverse effects on normal healing and on the natural defense against infectious disease.

Processed meats are unhealthy. Most contain poisonous chemicals and refined sugars. Many animals are given unhealthy grains, steroids, antibiotics and vaccines. Some animals are unhealthy when they are slaughtered. Human beings don't need to eat meats to be healthy. Meat is second hand food. When you eat meats you often eat the poisons concentrated in the meats. The same essential nutrients are found in fruits and vegetables.

It is a myth that people must eat animal products to get vitamin B12. Beneficial bacteria creates neurotransmitters and hormones like B12. Gorillas eat mainly raw green foods to maintain powerful muscles. Many great athletes are vegans.

The Vikings were a healthy race of people because they ate organic whole foods. They were not vegans or vegetarians. They ate fruits, herbs, vegetables, fish, fowl and other foods. Their water didn't contain chlorine and fluoride.

The wild game they ate wasn't vaccinated and fish didn't contain mercury. Animals weren't poisoned by growth steroids, genetically modified grains and antibiotics.

People can be healthy eating a vegan diet or eating like a Viking, but they cannot be healthy eating a lot of poisoned foods.

Cooking destroys many of the enzymes, vitamins and other nutrients. Vegans and vegetarians who eat a lot of cooked and poisoned foods suffer from chronic diseases.

You don't have to eat healthy foods all of the time to be healthy. There are degrees of health and fitness. The challenge you face is to decide how healthy and fit you want to be and then do what it takes to accomplish your personal goals. Life is a series of choices and experiences.

WEIGHT LOSS SOLUTION

*"Most obesity is the result of metabolic
disturbances, not over consumption of fat."*
–Dr. Robert C. Atkins

The word diet has more than one meaning. One definition is a special or limited selection of food or drink to bring about weight loss. The second definition is what a person usually eats or drinks.

When someone goes on a diet, they are usually referring to a temporary selection of food or drink. Restriction of certain food or drink can bring about weight loss, but as most people learn, the weight comes back when they return to their usual diet. The yo-yo effect is common and unhealthy.

There have been many diet books written throughout the years. Authors promise great results, but don't tell their readers when they go back to their regular diet, they will put the pounds back on.

There are diet programs which advertise special foods on the television every day. They make big promises about weight loss. These products may cause weight loss, but not good health.

*"Some animal studies show that sucrose is eight times
more addictive than cocaine." -Dr. Mark Hyman*

Most diet products contain harmful chemicals and refined sugars (sucrose, sorbitol, aspartame, etc.). These are the same things causing obesity and degenerative diseases. Protein drinks and energy bars are usually unhealthy. They are processed and unnatural.

102

Some diet products contain stimulants to speed up the metabolism. They may contain caffeine and other harmful drugs. These products are a temporary fix for a permanent dietary problem. Refined sugars and caffeine create a blood sugar-insulin roller coaster ride that can end in obesity, disease and death. High fructose corn syrup and artificial sweeteners are poisons which contribute to metabolic disorders, like hypoglycemia and diabetes.

The healthiest way to lose weight and keep it off is to give the body whole, nutrient-dense, organic foods and stop eating processed foods which cause metabolic imbalances.

Eat less and exercise more to lose weight and help speed up your metabolism. When we eat smaller meals our bodies can digest and use the nutrients more efficiently. You want to maintain a stable sugar-insulin balance by avoiding refined sugars and processed foods.

CLEANLINESS

To be healthy we need to cleanse the inside and outside of our bodies. Poor personal hygiene contributes to the spread of germs and a weak immune system. Washing our bodies, brushing our teeth, daily bowel movements and drinking enough water are vital to good health.

Drink plenty of water everyday to flush out heavy metals, man-made chemicals and human waste. Psyllium husks and fiber-dense foods help prevent constipation and acidosis.

Whenever you become ill, one of the best remedies is to rest, stop eating and drink a lot of clean water. The energy used to digest food will be used to fight germs and cleanse the body. As you detox, you may experience flu-like symptoms.

103

Drinking fresh green vegetable juices will help cleanse and alkalize the body, and supply essential nutrients. Foods like apples, raw apple cider vinegar, raw honey, garlic, cilantro are great for detoxing the body and helping white blood cells kill germs.

I recommend learning more about herbs. They can be used to help purify your body and kill harmful germs and parasites. Some of the most popular herbs for healing are goldenseal root, parsley, burdock root, ginger root, cayenne pepper, dandelion root, senna leaf, rhubarb root, licorice, clove, wormwood, echinacea and red clover blossom.

"Taking 400 mgs. of cilantro each day can remove
heavy metals from the body in just two weeks."
-Dr. Robert C. Atkins

ELECTROMAGNETIC RADIATION

Microwaves are a form of electromagnetic radiation. Microwave ovens, x-ray machines, cellular phones and electrical towers transmit harmful radiation. Invisible electrical waves damage blood cells and tissues which can lead to fungal infection and tumors.

Televisions, computers and modems also transmit harmful radiation. When people go to the mountains they usually feel better because they escape most electromagnetic fields (smart meters, towers and other sources of electricity).

For thousands of years human beings have walked barefoot or wore shoes with leather soles. Rubber soled shoes prevent the body from grounding. Our world and our bodies are electromagnetic. Walking barefoot is health enhancing.

SUNLIGHT

Sunlight is a vital nutrient for most plants and animals. Human beings need ultraviolet radiation to create Vitamin D. Our bodies depend on this hormone to function properly. A lack of Vitamin D has been linked to many chronic diseases. Most sunscreens contain poisonous chemicals and block out healthy UV rays. Sunbathing for 15 minutes per day will contribute to a healthier body. Use common sense and avoid sunburn by limiting time in the sun or covering your body.

EXERCISE

"Physical fitness is not only one of the most important keys to a healthy body, it is the basis of a dynamic and creative intellectual activity." - John F. Kennedy

Exercise is vital to good health. To have strong muscles and bones you must use them. Bones, ligaments, tendons and muscles become bigger with movement and pressure.

Oxygen is delivered to cells throughout the body by the bloodstream. Arteries and veins are the major blood vessels. The heart pumps blood away from the heart and it returns by way of the veins. The veins require movement to function at their best.

Exercise is activity that helps the body cleanse out poisons, take in more oxygen and circulate the blood faster. Working up a sweat can help release poisons, but it also creates a loss of essential minerals. Drink plenty of clean water to avoid dehydration.

Walking, running, working, gardening, dancing or playing sports are all good for getting your metabolism and circulation going faster. Aerobic exercises, when done properly, help to strengthen the heart and other muscles. If you need or want bigger and stronger muscles, then lifting weights are the way to go.

We don't need to lift weights, run or vigorously exercise three times a week, but we do want to be active. Many people have back problems because their stomach and back muscles are out of shape. Some people drop dead from heart attacks while appearing to be healthy. A person can be physically fit and still be unhealthy.

REST AND RELAXATION

Too much stress can kill you. Stress is tension. Relaxation is a state of the body when you have a small amount of muscle tension. Relaxed sleeping is vital for maintaining good health and energy. Sleep deprivation causes the brain to malfunction.

Stress is not a bad thing. The problem is too much tension for too long. Going through the day with too much tension uses up valuable energy. If your body is run down, you have less energy to control germs. When you learn to stay more relaxed, you will have more energy and be able to sleep better at night.

LOVE AND COMPANIONSHIP

"Without love, life seems absurd and not worth living."
-Linda Jane Ellison

106

We all want to feel important and loved. Loneliness is a painful feeling. Receiving and giving affection is important to our spiritual well being. It's human nature to seek approval and attention. We are spirit beings inside temporary bodies.

"You know you're in love when you can't fall asleep because reality is finally better than your dreams." -Dr. Seuss

GOD, PRAYER AND FAITH

"I know the world is ruled by infinite intelligence. There is a great directing head of people and things. A supreme being who looks after the destinies of the world."
-Thomas Edison

Faith in a loving God can be one of the most comforting beliefs someone can have. Counting your blessings every day and appreciating your life is health enhancing.

When you give thanks for your blessings, you visualize them. When you pray for others or for good things to happen, you use positive words and imagery. Prayer can be a powerful form of positive thinking.

Human beings are controlled by beliefs and emotions. Many people put their faith in organized religions or scientific theories. No one knows for sure how this world and human beings came into existence.

.

PURPOSE

To live a fuller life we need a sense of purpose. We all need someone to love and something to live for. Human beings are goal striving creatures.

Goals give us something to focus on and work towards. It's exciting to go after a challenging goal. Life is about much more than the pursuit of money or happiness. Helping others is one of the most joyful things you can do.

"The purpose of life
is not to be happy.
It is to be useful,
to be honorable,
to be compassionate,
to have it make some
difference that you have
lived and lived well."

-Ralph Waldo Emerson

"From the hardest fought battles
come the sweetest victories."
-Anonymous

SUMMARY

1. Your body is like an automobile with a computer system. To maintain a well running body you must give it the nutrients it needs and stop putting in the wrong fuel.
2. The human body, including the brain cannot function properly while being poisoned or lacking essential minerals.
3. Processed foods lack essential nutrients and contain poisons.
4. The natural, organic, primitive diet is the best.
5. Whatever you breathe, eat, drink, or think affects your body chemistry.
6. The body needs to be continually cleansed of harmful substances.
7. Drinking organic green juices is one the best ways to alkalize the bloodstream and supply needed nutrients.
8. You must relax and get enough rest or your energy level and white blood cell count will go down and then you become vulnerable to germs and the viruses they excrete.
9. Human bodies are electrical machines which convert sunlight, oxygen, water and minerals into electrical energy.
10. Start taking action to create a healthy body.

*"I shall pass through
this world but once. Any good
therefore that I can do, or any
kindness that I can show to any
human being, let me do it now.
Let me not defer nor neglect it,
for I shall not pass this way again."*

- Stephen Grellet

SECTION THREE

How To
Develop Self-Control

*"Order and simplification
are the first steps toward
mastery of a subject."*

-Thomas Mann

*"Common sense
is not so common."*

-Voltaire

CHAPTER NINE

Mental Healing

*"The major hypoglycemia symptoms are mental
confusion, emotional instability, low energy,
and neurotic and psychotic behavior."*
-Dr. Paavo Airola

I worked with a man named Stan. When he was a boy he
suffered from mental illness. His parents took him to many
doctors. The doctors said he was manic depressive,
schizophrenic and suffering from chemical imbalances in his
brain. They also told his parents there is no cure for his mental
problems.

Stan was treated with prescription drugs and
psychotherapy. He continued to have mood swings and
hallucinations.

Eventually Stan's parents found a doctor who cured him.
The doctor told them, his mental problems are caused by
refined sugar and caffeine. The brain cannot function properly
while it's being drugged.

When Stan stopped eating and drinking things that
contained those stimulating poisons, his mood swings and
irrational behavior went away. He was able to relax during the
day and sleep at night because his brain chemistry was
changed.

Stan became well because his parents found a doctor with the correct knowledge to solve his mental problems. Stan escaped a mental health trap.

Drugs and talk therapy could never have cured Stan. They cannot cure other people with mental problems caused by chemical poisoning, lack of essential nutrients or sleep deprivation.

THE MIND

Webster's New World Dictionary defines the word mind as: memory, opinion, the seat of consciousness, intellect, spirit, reason; sanity.

The word mind is used as a figure of speech. No one literally loses their mind, goes out of their mind or finds peace of mind. We often use the words mind or mental when referring to how the brain is functioning.

The mind's eye is a metaphor for the imagination. Imagination is defined as the ability to create ideas and mental images. It's a natural function of the brain and spirit.

The conscious and subconscious minds are metaphors. They refer to the abilities and processes of the brain and spirit.

You aren't a mind, body and spirit. You are a spirit being in an electronic body, with a computer-like brain.

BRAIN-ALTERING DRUGS

Mental illness is a physical problem. Many people are unaware that caffeine, refined sugars and other chemicals poison the brain and cause it to malfunction. **They don't realize how much their diet affects their mental health.**

114

Antidepressants and tranquilizing drugs can create the illusion of a cure by controlling symptoms. They can also cause depression, psychotic behavior and suicide. Many violent crimes are committed by people while under the influence of prescription drugs. **Most psychiatrists have little or no training in nutrition and the proper care of the human brain.** They are usually trained to use drugs and talk therapy to control symptoms.

"Only approximately six percent of the graduating physicians in the U.S. have training in nutrition." -Dr. Ray D. Strand

I know a woman who went to the doctor because she felt depressed. It never occurred to her that depression could be caused by her unhealthy diet. Her doctor prescribed an antidepressant drug. The drug poisoned her brain and affected her ability to feel emotions.

Twenty years later she was still taking prescription drugs. Her diet didn't change and her symptoms never went away. She wasn't cured, she was only drugged. She was caught in a mental health trap.

I know a man who suffers from schizophrenia and bipolar disorder symptoms. Caffeine and refined sugar cause a brain chemistry imbalance and sleep deprivation, which results in his mental problems.

He was first diagnosed with mental illness when he was 17 and has been taking prescription drugs for over 35 years. At one time he was taking six different drugs.

Tranquilizers counteract the stimulants and help his brain relax. Sleep deprivation can cause him to become psychotic and violent.

He has seen many doctors through the years. They have been unable to heal him with prescription drugs and talk therapy. He is in a vicious cycle of drug addiction and chemical dependency.

Chemicals in our diet can cause depression, mood swings, hallucinations, sleep deprivation and brain chemistry imbalances.

SLEEP DEPRIVATION

Chronic insomnia is a serious problem. The brain is an electrical and chemical machine that must be recharged by sleeping. The spirit also needs rest. When the brain is stimulated and poisoned by chemicals, it's impossible to relax and sleep well.

Sleep deprivation causes neurotic and psychotic behavior. If you don't get enough sleep you will eventually become depressed, irrational and insane.

Anyone who goes without sleep will eventually hallucinate, and have the same psychotic symptoms, as a person labeled schizophrenic. Hearing voices and seeing things are some of the symptoms of sleep deprivation.

A lack of sleep causes children to become cranky and irrational. Some children require a nap in the afternoon and plenty of sleep at night for their brains to function properly.

Many people are unaware of all of the chemicals in processed foods which affect their ability to think clearly and sleep soundly. Using poisons, such as alcohol and other drugs to relax and sleep have negative effects on the brain.

BRAIN CHEMISTRY

Many people get hooked on refined sugar and caffeine when they are children. Their brains are on a roller coaster ride of high and low blood sugar. Some autism spectrum disorders, such as ADD or ADHD can be caused by these chemicals.

People act differently when under the influence of prescription drugs, caffeine, refined sugars or alcohol. It's not a coincidence that many homeless and mentally ill people are hooked on coffee, sodas or alcohol.

When fitness expert Jack Lalanne was a boy, he suffered from mental illness. He almost killed his brother while under the influence of refined sugar. Lalanne admitted he was a sugaraholic and unhealthy. **For over fifty years he warned people about the dangers of eating processed foods.**

Dr. Paavo Airola wrote a book called *Hypoglycemia; A Better Approach.* His revolutionary book exposes how many mental disorders, such as depression, bipolar and schizophrenia are caused by chemicals in our diets. Dr. Airola has helped thousands of people become well.

"Such knowledge may also give us clues as to why so many of us become schizophrenics, alcoholics, tobacco-coffee-coke-drug-addicts and suicide victims."
-Dr. Paavo Airola

117

PARASITES AND MENTAL ILLNESS

"Over two billion people suffer from parasites."
-World Health Organization

Parasites cause mental illness. The syphilis bacteria causes insanity by destroying brain cells. Worms (trichinosis) in the brain also causes insanity. Candida albicans, aspergillus, penicillum, cryptococcus and other types of fungi can get in the brain and destroy brain cells. **The fungus colonizes to form plaques, sclerosis, tumors, etc.**

Some cases of depression, bipolar disorder and schizophrenia are caused by fungus. Fungus can excrete powerful viruses, which kill brain cells and cause insanity. **Rabies symptoms are a good example of brain damage caused by fungi and the viruses they excrete.**

TRAUMATIC EXPERIENCES

"Trauma; a bodily injury of shock or an emotional shock, often having lasting psychic effect."
- Webster's New World Dictionary

The human body is an electromagnetic machine. An exciting experience causes the brain to generate more electricity and release hormones. The brain and nervous system can be shocked into trance states.

Sometimes people will have no conscious memory of a traumatic experience. They may block out the memory to cope with the pain. Some traumatic experiences have lasting effect.

118

A highly emotional person sometimes acts irrational because the same brain he or she uses to reason with is under the influence of powerful chemicals called hormones. When our brains are under the influence of man-made chemicals or hormones, it's much harder to tell the difference between reality and imaginary images. Many times we react to our own mental pictures as if they are reality.

TRAUMA BASED MIND CONTROL

People sometimes go into a trance state when their attention is focused on one thing. A good example of this phenomenon is the trances created while watching television or movies. While in a trance state the brain can be programmed much easier.

Animals and human beings are sometimes trained by creating trauma. Pimps use abuse and drugs to program their slaves. Military drill instructors deliberately create confusion, fear, pain and stress to create submissive followers.

In the 1950s, the CIA created MK Ultra Programs which used trauma based mind control techniques. Thousands of people have been unwilling or unknowing victims of their experiments.

Severe abuse, electric shock, hypnosis and drugs can be used to create trances, psychotic behaviors and identity confusion. Disassociative Identity Disorder (Multiple Personality Disorder) can be created by repeated abuse and programming of the brain.

MENTAL HEALTHCARE

Mental healthcare is imperfect. Some elements of mental healthcare are good, while others are harmful. **Psychiatrists and other therapists suffer from anxiety, confusion and bad habits just like everyone else.**

In 1952, the American Psychiatric Association (APA) first published the Diagnostic and Statistical Manual of Mental Disorders. Since then, the APA has gradually added new disorders with each publication.

Psychiatrists classify abnormal behavior as a neurosis or a psychosis. A psychosis is a state of thinking in which the person may lose contact with reality. A neurosis is characterized by anxiety, compulsions and phobias.

Some of the other symptoms are trance states, identity and gender confusion, delusions, hallucinations and bizarre behavior. The symptoms are given disorder names.

Neurotic and psychotic behavior can be created by irrational thoughts and beliefs. The hypochondriac is a good example of how an uncontrolled imagination can cause anxiety and eventually illness.

In the past, schizophrenic symptoms such as hallucinations and loss of contact with reality were sometimes called a nervous breakdown. The brain and nervous system break down and malfunction.

Psychiatrists don't know how to solve many mental problems. They have used electroshock, drugs, talk therapy and even lobotomies to control patients who suffered from malfunctioning brains or demonic possession.

Electroshock therapy is performed by electrocuting the patient until the patient becomes more docile. Electrocuting the brain cannot solve a mental problem. Trauma based mind control also uses electrical shocking to create altered states. Drug therapy is also used to create docile patients and stop symptoms. Children diagnosed with autism disorders are sometimes drugged for the same purpose.

Talk therapy such as psychoanalysis is a form of mind control. Therapists have their own opinion about each disorder and the treatment for it. Talk therapy sometimes causes more confusion and codependency.

Lobotomies were also performed to create docile patients. The procedure was usually done by inserting a sharp object, such as an ice pick into the brain through the eye socket. The procedure was popular at one time, but it caused severe brain damage to patients.

"Those who can make you believe absurdities can make you commit atrocities." -Voltaire

PSYCHIATRY

Psychology is a science dealing with mental, emotional, and behavioral processes. It's complex and confusing. A great deal of modern psychology is based on myths and unproven ideas.

Sigmund Freud is considered by many to be the father of modern psychiatry. Some people believe his theories are proven facts. Many of his theorics were created while he was under the influence of drugs.

Freud was a cocaine user and had many other destructive habits. He promoted cocaine as a cure for many mental problems. Freud may not have understood how diet and drugs affect the brain.

PSYCHOTHERAPY

Psychotherapy is a treatment which involves dwelling on past experiences. It's usually expensive and painful. The therapy often helps to reinforce unwanted thought and behavior patterns.

Ivan Pavlov is famous for his work with dogs and automatic responses, called classical conditioning. Through repetition he trained his dogs to associate food with the sound of a bell. Pavlov knew how to create habit patterns and break them as well.

When Pavlov wanted to break an automatic response, he stopped reinforcing the pattern. He interrupted the pattern over and over, until it faded away.

Many psychiatrists diagnose their patients and tell them they have *incurable* disorders. When patients believe their mental problems are incurable they become trapped.

Some therapists cause feelings of inferiority by setting unrealistic standards. They tell their patients they are abnormal. The word normal means to conform with an accepted standard.

"Why fit in when you were born to stand out?"
-Dr. Seuss

SPIRITS

"We are not human beings on a spiritual journey. We are spiritual beings on a human journey." -Steven R. Covey

Spirits are *physical* beings which usually can't be seen with the naked eye. They are as physical as oxygen, microorganisms and radio waves.

Telescopes and microscopes help us see physical things we cannot see with the naked eye. In some ways, we are handicapped by our eyesight.

Every spirit which enters a body already has unique qualities. Most parents will agree each one of their children had a different personality at birth. My son and daughter are two very different spirit beings.

If you examine a litter of puppies, you will see the different qualities shortly after birth. Anyone who has owned more than one dog knows each dog is unique.

When I was a boy, I had a pony and a chicken who became best friends. The pony allowed the chicken to ride and sleep on her back. They communicated with each other using a mysterious language.

John Growney is a rodeo stock contractor and owner of the famous bucking bull named Red Rock. John is aware of the different personalities of each bull.

Red Rock liked people, but didn't like other bulls. He would allow children to ride him, but not bull riders who attempted to ride him at rodeos.

123

John can't prove it, but he suspects the spirit inside Red Rock may have been a bull rider in a previous life. Red Rock was more than just another bull. He was a member of John's family.

MENTAL TELEPATHY

The brain can transmit and receive electrical thought waves. Prayer and mental telepathy are the same phenomenon. When you pray, you are sending out physical thought waves. We all have a *sixth sense*, in which we transmit and receive thoughts.

Ideas can come from outside our physical brains and flash into our awareness. The brain is similar to a computer which can log onto the Internet. The information is invisible to the naked eye. We can communicate with what has been called God, the collective consciousness and infinite intelligence.

A computer has the ability to manage information. It can store, receive, transmit and process data like the human brain. Computers and brains are both programmable machines which respond to specific sets of instructions. Human beings are programmed to believe and behave in certain ways.

Spirits can communicate with us using physical thought waves. They can talk to you even if you are in the jungle or the middle of the ocean.

"My brain is only a receiver. In the Universe there is a core from which we obtain knowledge, strength and inspiration."
-Nikola Tesla, inventor

124

Cellphones are a good example of how mental telepathy works. In the 1960s the television series *Star Trek* used cellphone devices called communicators. Back then the idea seemed absurd. We now take this technology for granted. Invisible sound waves are transported around the world in seconds. These electrical energy waves are transmitted and received by our phones. The electrical waves are physical energy.

A television is another example of how invisible energy is transmitted through the air by converting light rays into electrical signals. Radios also receive electromagnetic waves which are sent out at different frequencies (cycles per unit of time).

Microwave Auditory Effect (MAE) technology is used to transmit thoughts (physical sound waves) into the human brain. The MAE system is called MEDUSA (Mob Excess Deterrent Using Silent Audio) and is intended to remotely, temporarily incapacitate people.

THE LAW OF ATTRACTION

Some people believe there is a secret way to become healthy and successful without effort. The biggest misunderstanding about the law of attraction is the belief that you control all of your experiences, by your thoughts. This unrealistic idea includes controlling other people. How is that possible if everyone else is controlling all of their experiences too? Many unrealistic ideas are received from deceiving spirits by way of mental telepathy.

The definition of attract is to draw to itself or oneself. Magnets can repel or attract using an invisible power. The brain is an electromagnetic computer and has the power to attract ideas.

The brain has the ability to find or create ideas which can solve problems or achieve goals. When ideas come they should be written down as soon as possible, so they aren't forgotten. Songwriters, inventors and what some people call geniuses are aware that ideas pop into their heads.

Thomas Edison and Nikola Tesla used this natural ability of the human brain (transmitting and receiving thoughts) to find answers to their questions.

The process is similar to trying to remember someone's name. You must want to remember and then tell your brain to search for the name. The name can come to you hours later when you have stopped trying to remember. Your desire, focused attention and effort are important.

SUPERNATURAL MIND CONTROL

"Hell is empty and all the devils are here."
-William Shakespeare

The definition of the word demon is an evil spirit. **The word possess means to take control of someone or something.** Evil entities can possess human and animal bodies.

Demons are parasitic creatures which cause mental problems. They have always influenced human behavior using deceptive methods.

The word evil means anything which causes harm. People are desensitized to many things that are evil. Demons have trained people to believe many lies and desire things which are destructive and dangerous.

We have been manipulated by supernatural beings for thousands of years and much of the evil that people call "human nature" is really demonic nurturing.

Witchcraft is a religion in which followers use words and rituals to contact spirits and gain power. Most men and women who practice witchcraft keep their beliefs and behaviors hidden. Some cast spells, evoke demons and perform rituals which involve cannibalism or sexual abuse.

Mental telepathy, television, radio, books, movies and other methods are used to train and control the minds of people. Every man, woman and child are being influenced by evil spirits. Demons feed off our energy and appear to enjoy our suffering.

Demons can take complete or partial control of the brain. The serial killer Jeffrey Dahmer is a good example of complete demonic control. Jeffrey was obsessed with torture, rape, murder, dismemberment, necrophilia and cannibalism.

Most serial killers, psychopaths and satanists look and act respectable when in public. They enjoy deceiving and abusing people. Some devil worshipers enjoy flaunting their faith.

Demons are like backseat drivers. They try to influence what we think and do. Some enter and leave bodies in the same manner you would enter and leave an automobile. More than one entity can be inside a body at the same time.

Demons are not metaphors or symbols. Many people are aware spirits communicate with them. Some believe they have a good angel or a family member watching over them but they don't want to believe evil spirits exist.

Dr. M. Scott Peck is a psychiatrist who became convinced demons are real and they cause many mental disorders. He tried to get the American Psychiatric Association to recognize evil spirits as *one* cause of mental illness.

Many mental problems are caused by demons. They can cause psychotic thinking and behavior. Some obsessive compulsive disorders are demonic temptations. The word tempt means to compel or entice, to do something.

The uncontrolled repetitive cussing and perverted behavior of some people with Tourette syndrome (TS) is a good example of demonic influence. Doctors don't know the cause of TS. They use drugs to alter brain chemistry and try to manage symptoms.

Some of the symptoms of TS are uncontrolled body movements, grunting, barking, hitting oneself, indecent touching of themselves or others, vulgar gesturing, altering of the voice and shouting swear words.

If TS is only a brain problem, why is the repetitive uncontrolled behavior often morally bad or harmful?

Many Christians want a good spirit to enter their bodies. They believe a spirit or ghost enters their bodies and then they are able to speak in different languages.

"And they were all filled with the Holy Ghost, and began to speak with other tongues, as the spirit gave them utterance."
-Acts 2:4, King James Version

"For we wrestle not against flesh and blood, but against principalities, against powers, against the rulers of the darkness of this world, against spiritual wickedness in high places." -Ephesians 6:12, King James Version

128

The spirit realm is a *physical* realm. The definition of a spirit is the life principle in human beings and other animals. A spirit is also defined as a supernatural entity such as an angel. Some psychics become possessed by spirits or communicate with them using mental telepathy. Many people who practice voodoo want to be filled with a supernatural entity. Satanic rituals are also performed to communicate with entities and sometimes become possessed by them.

Newborn babies and people of all ages can become possessed by demons. Many entertainers communicate with spirits and allow them to enter their bodies before performing.

Jim Morrison, Jimmy Hendrix, Robin Williams, Michael Jackson, Denzel Washington, Beyonce, Oprah and many other entertainers have admitted spirits *take over* their bodies while performing.

Demonic voices can cause people to believe they are going insane. Mike Tyson believes he has been tormented by demons. They create mental confusion.

Evil spirits want us to hurt ourselves and each other. They cause people to commit suicide and violent acts. The leading causes of suicide are demonic voices and pain. Multiple personality disorder and gender confusion can also be caused by demons.

I talked to a woman named Mary about her childhood. She said her stepmother abused her and her brother. One day she held her younger brother's hand over the stove fire and burned him. Mary told me, "I believe demons are real because I saw the look in my stepmother's eyes when the demon would take over her body."

I remember reading about a mother who killed all five of her children. She said an evil being took over her body. The judge and jury didn't want to believe demons are real.

Whenever a man or woman kills their family and then commits suicide, drugs and demons are usually involved. Demons can make us say and do harmful things.

"Sexual predators have demons that seek out jobs around children." -Senator Charles Schumer

Demons can cause people to lie, cheat and steal. They torment human beings by telling them they are worthless and deserve to die.

Demons cause unrealistic thinking and destructive behavior. People with anorexia or bulimia are being manipulated by evil spirits. Those people may overeat, purge, excessively exercise, use laxatives and starve their bodies.

Anorexia and bulimia are disease names given to behaviors which involve self-abuse. People with eating disorders sometimes have other destructive behaviors such as cutting, head banging, burning, limb amputation (transabled people), hair pulling and bone breaking.

I met a woman named Lani who became addicted to heroin. She told me voices tormented her day and night. Demons persuaded her to use heroin to escape the voices she believed were her own.

She said using heroin is an evil trap. She now realizes supernatural beings are physical and some of them are causing people to abuse themselves and others.

Most of the demons' power comes from deception and keeping us confused with incorrect knowledge. The definition of the word confusion is lack of understanding and a state of chaos. It's vital for us to become aware of how demons manipulate us. Prayer is a powerful weapon. We can pray for God's help and for others who are deceived. We can command demons to shut up and leave using the power of God and our spoken words. Evil spirits can come back and must be resisted each time.

SPIRITS AND RELIGION

People living thousands of years ago were communicating with supernatural beings. They have been called gods, goddesses, angels, demons, guides, ghosts, spirits, and aliens. Primitive people living in all parts of the world communicated with them. These entities can appear, disappear, shape shift and enter the bodies of people and animals.

Shamans and other religious leaders have always known spirits are *physical* beings. These entities influence world leaders. Some people willingly become possessed by them during secret ceremonies.

Religious ceremonies, seances, witchcraft, prayer, Ouija boards and psychics are some of the methods used to communicate with supernatural beings.

The Sumerians, Babylonians, Egyptians, Hebrews, Greeks and Romans believed in entities who could look like people or other creatures. It seems these beings have always influenced our religious beliefs throughout recorded history.

Our beliefs greatly affect our perception. Some people believe life is an illusion. The word illusion means a false idea or conception. It also means an unreal or misleading image.

Human beings believe many false ideas and are deceived by misleading images. Some people believe evil supernatural beings aren't real until they personally encounter one.

According to the Bible, Job 1:6-12, God, Satan and other angels work together to test the spirit beings who are in human bodies. We are rewarded and punished by them.

The word angel means a spirit believed to act as an attendant, agent, or messenger of God. Some people believe angels watch, guard, tempt, torture and help mankind. They also believe the angels monitor our thoughts and actions 24 hours a day.

If the Bible is correct then we are spirits, living in a world ruled by God and Satan. We are here to participate in a contest between good and evil. We enter human bodies and then each one of us plays different roles. It's all part of a learning, growing, testing and sorting process.

Maybe, we are like the puppet Pinocchio. He had to develop a conscience and prove he could be truthful, brave and unselfish. He developed good character after making many wrong choices. His life was an adventure with a series of challenging learning experiences. An adventure is a daring, hazardous and sometimes romantic experience.

"It's not whether you win or lose,
it's how you play the game."
-Grantland Rice

132

NEAR DEATH EXPERIENCES

A near death experience is an unusual experience which occurs when a person is near death or temporarily dead and is resuscitated.

I lived across the street from a man named Steve. He told me how he was kicked in the head by a horse and died. Steve remembers the ambulance ride to the hospital and how he could hear and see the paramedics even though they believed he was dead.

Steve saw a white light and a voice spoke to him saying, "You have to go back into your body. You have things you must do. You are going to be alright."

I have researched temporary death experiences and many of the stories aren't positive. Some spirits hover over their bodies, while others seem to take a journey into the spirit realm. People are known to see and hear horrible things during that time.

One man I talked to said he had heart surgery and died on the operating table. He told me he went to a hellish place and felt thankful to enter his body again.

It's impossible to prove there are heavenly and hellish places in the spirit world, but millions of people swear their out-of-body experiences were real.

"If you want to find the secrets of the universe,
think in terms of energy, frequency and vibration."
-Nikola Tesla

133

"The major hypoglycemia symptoms are mental confusion, emotional instability, low energy, and neurotic and psychotic behavior." -Dr. Paavo Airola

SUMMARY

1. Refined sugars, caffeine and other chemicals can cause mental illness.
2. Mental illness is physical illness.
3. The word mind is a metaphor.
4. Mental healthcare is imperfect. Some elements are good, while others are harmful. Psychiatry is based on many incorrect theories and myths.
5. Prescription drugs and talk therapy can't cure mental problems caused by diet, drugs, sleep deprivation or demons.
6. Parasites can cause mental illness.
7. Antidepressants and other mind-altering drugs are dangerous. While under the influence of these drugs, people sometimes commit violent acts and suicide.
8. You are a spirit in an electromagnetic body.
9. Thoughts are physical. The brain has the ability to transmit and receive electrical thought waves.
10. Prayer and mental telepathy are a physical phenomenon and a sixth sense.
11. Demons are physical beings. There appears to be a contest or battle between good and evil spirits.
12. Demons have been practicing mind control techniques for thousands of years. They are our invisible enemies.
13. Demons can be cast out of people. Praying for guidance and protection can help.
14. Start taking action to create good mental health.

CHAPTER TEN

Self-Control Skills

*"There never has been, and cannot be, a good
life without self-control." -Leo Tolstoy*

Stress is physical tension. Tension is tightness in muscles and
increased brain and nervous system stimulation. The brain and
nervous system operate using electricity and chemicals.

Relaxation is a state of the body where there is a small
amount of tension in the muscles and brain waves are slowed
down. When brain waves are slower and muscles are relaxed,
there is more self-control and a feeling called peace of mind.

As the brain receives more stimulation, the brain waves
speed up and create tension in the body. The more excited a
person becomes the more out of control or automatic the
behavior may become.

Learning to relax your muscles is one of the greatest skills
you can develop. All great performers relax and focus on the
job at hand. They learn to use the right amount of tension to
perform at their best.

To be able to perform well on and off the field, you must learn to relax and control your thinking. When you learn how to use the right amount of muscle tension and concentrate on the present moment, you will be able to control your emotions much better.

Many people go through the day using too much effort. They are overly tense, as if they are ready to run or fight. Going through the day in a fight or flight state of tension is exhausting. In most situations staying relaxed will help you react faster and make better decisions.

MEDITATION

"Meditation is a practice in which an individual trains the "mind" or induces a mode of consciousness."
-Wikipedia, meditation

The definition of meditate is to focus your attention or think deeply. Concentrating on one thing helps to alter brain waves and create emotional states. Meditation can also be used for mental rehearsal to improve skills or alter beliefs and behaviors.

You don't need to sit in a lotus position, touch your fingers together or say the word Om to relax your brain. The key is concentrating on one thing which relaxes the brain. Focusing your attention and controlling your words and imagery will relax your brain.

Your brain operates at different frequencies (cycles per second) while awake and asleep. Brain cells interact by electrical impulses. Your brain waves can be measured using an electroencephalograph.

136

The brain regulates body temperature, digestion, heart beat, breathing, fight or flight response, emotions and other autonomic functions. Controlling how you stimulate or relax your brain is the key to creating the emotions you desire.

RELAXATION BASICS

Remind yourself that words and images can create muscle tension or relaxation.

Relaxation is the absence of tension in your muscles. It will happen when you concentrate on one thing which slows down electrical brainwaves and releases tension.

Practice the relaxation exercise everyday. You will develop the skill of mental focusing and releasing tension. Make a recording of this exercise or have someone read the words to you slowly and softly. Eventually you will develop the ability to release tension quickly and maintain a more relaxed mental attitude during the day. You will also remember what to say to yourself and not need a recording or friend to guide you.

Go into a quiet room, lie down and close your eyes. You don't want any distractions. Closing your eyes will reduce brain stimulation caused by images. Your goal is to control your words and imagination. Practice is the key to success.

RELAXATION EXERCISE

Concentrate on my voice. Take a deep, slow breath. Breathe from your diaphragm and as you exhale let out a sigh. Take another deep breath and focus on breathing slowly. Now, take five breaths as you count from five to one. Breathe in slowly and out slowly.

137

Now, tighten the muscles in your feet. Hold the tension for two seconds then let go of the tension. Now, tighten the muscles in your legs.

Hold for two seconds then let the muscles relax. Now, tighten the muscles in your stomach. Hold for two seconds then relax. Now, tighten your back muscles then let the muscles relax.

Now, take three deep, slow breaths and sigh when you exhale. Let go of the tension inside your body. You are safe now, you can let go of your tension.

Now, tighten your chest muscles and then let them go. Now, tighten your arms and hands and then let the muscles relax. Now, tighten your jaw muscles and then let them go limp. Now, tighten the muscles in your forehead and then let them relax. Take three deep slow breaths and sigh as you exhale.

Become aware of how you feel at this moment. The next time you want to be relaxed, the way you are now, say the word relax. The word relax will trigger this feeling.

Now, I am going to count from one to five. When I get to five you will be wide awake and feel good. You will want to release tension by doing this exercise every day. The best time is in the afternoon or before bedtime.

One...two...three...four...five. Open your eyes.

EMOTIONS

Emotions are strong feelings caused by electrical and chemical reactions in the body. The release of hormones and electrical impulses within the brain and nervous system cause pleasurable or painful sensations.

Emotions are created when the brain becomes stimulated by one or more of the five senses (sight, touch, taste, smell or hearing). When our brains are relaxed we show very little emotional reaction. Emotions are also created by how you use your body. The brain and facial muscles are wired together and automatically trigger certain emotions like anger, fear, sadness and happiness. If you smile and walk as if you are happy, that behavior helps to create a feeling of happiness.

When your muscles become tense, your emotional state changes. Your muscles affect your attitude. It's almost impossible to stay depressed if you smile, laugh and visualize pleasant experiences.

PAIN AND PLEASURE

People are controlled by their beliefs and feelings of pain and pleasure. We usually try to avoid painful experiences and seek pleasurable ones.

Happiness is the feeling of pleasure which comes and goes. It's unrealistic to believe you can feel good all of the time. Happiness is a feeling which can be created by chemicals, experiencing something you enjoy or visualizing a pleasant experience.

If you want to feel good more often you need to control your self-talk and imagery. Whatever you imagine or say to yourself affects your brain and nervous system. Emotions are created by *real or imagined* experiences. Your words and images can be your best friend or worst enemy.

Become more aware of how the radio, television, movies, songs, books, demons and other people influence your feelings.

139

The emotions of anger, love, fear and even sadness can be pleasurable or painful. Human beings can be trained to associate pleasure with pain. Some people like the feeling of pain.

Hate or anger can be positive when overcoming an abusive person or a drug addiction. Love can be negative when a person continues a destructive relationship with a person or drug because they love the pleasure. Fear can be a negative or positive emotion. It can help save your life, or stop you from living a full life.

WORD IMAGERY THINKING

Your brain is like a DVD player. You can create the emotions you desire. If you put a funny movie in the DVD player, you wouldn't expect that movie to make you feel sad.

The music in a movie, song or commercial is used to create emotions. A good example is the movie *Jaws*. Music was used to excite the viewers.

You can choose which memories to play or which mental pictures you want to create. Thinking is the process of imagining experiences and focusing on ideas. When you think, you use words and images. The mental pictures automatically create emotions, as if the experience is actually happening. The imagination is your power and ability to create ideas and mental pictures.

Webster's New World Dictionary defines the word wit as the powers of thinking. To remember how your brain and spirit communicate, think of the word wit as an acronym, which stands for *Word Imagery Thinking.*

EMOTION EXERCISE

To better understand how emotions are created, practice this exercise at least 10 times..

First, close your eyes and visualize a happy experience from your past. Focus your attention on the images as if you are watching a movie. Tell yourself the experience is beautiful. Eventually you will create feelings that are similar to those in the past.

Next, visualize a traumatic memory. The more vivid the images are, the faster you will create sad or fearful feelings. Tell yourself the experience is painful. Eventually you will create painful feelings.

Now, focus your attention on your breathing. Tell yourself to breathe slowly and deeply ten times. As you concentrate on the present moment you will not visualize painful or pleasurable memories. You will be controlling your words and imagery and creating peaceful feelings.

You can create happy or sad feelings by remembering past experiences or visualizing possible future experiences.

CAN TECHNIQUE

Now, think of the word can. The word can is an acronym for *Change Attention Now*. The word attention means focusing on something or someone. It also means mental concentration.

When you want to change your feelings, change what you are paying attention to. Tell yourself to stop and then choose what you want to focus your attention on. Many people are unaware how little they are controlling their thinking.

When we try to not think about something we are actually focusing our attention on it. If I tell you don't think about pink elephants, I'm causing you to visualize them.

141

When a person tries not to stutter he is focusing on stuttering. The person who tries to fall asleep causes the brain to stay tense. People who dwell on past traumas reinforce the memories and feelings each time.

Cravings are temporary feelings and desires. One of the keys to stopping unwanted feelings and behaviors is to change what you are thinking about. Don't fight the cravings, that keeps you focusing your attention on the same thing. Instead focus your attention on something else and your feelings and desire will change automatically.

Ninety percent of what we feel, think and do is done habitually. Our brains are trained to react automatically. The brain is a habit machine. The way we walk, talk and do many things is done with little conscious thinking.

When athletes are playing in the zone they are actually in a very focused state and performing the way they have trained their brains to automatically react. An athlete wants to be in a focused state where the brain takes over and performs the split second reactions.

A good example of this is how a bull rider must react by reflexes because there is no time to consciously think. The person with habitual unwanted feelings or behaviors is often reacting the way the brain has been trained.

Pavlov's dogs reacted in an automatic way because of previous training. One key to gaining more control of our emotions is to interrupt the automatic habit patterns and retrain the brain.

Focusing on the present moment is vital to being able to react appropriately to the present moment. Sometimes people drive to or from work and don't remember driving. They may be watching the road while visualizing something else.

Listening to the radio causes the brain to visualize. The words of a song can also trigger memories. Songwriters use words and music to capture your attention. They want you to create mental pictures and powerful emotions. The brain controls the autonomic nervous system. Most of the functions of the body are done automatically. We automatically memorize and visualize. The brain is wired to create mental pictures and emotions when stimulated by words.

Traumatic and sad memories can be left in the past when you take control of your imagination. The past loses its power when you stop visualizing past experiences, and focus your attention on the present moment.

Using the CAN technique will help you interrupt fear, worry, cravings and obsessive compulsive thinking. Changing what you are visualizing, watching or listening to, will change your emotions and desires.

Demons can talk to us and put images in our brains. You can command demons to shut up and go away and tell your brain to stop the mental pictures.

Practice is the key to developing skills and reinforcing good and bad habits. Practice the CAN technique everyday and you will develop more control of your imagination and emotions.

PERFECTION AND EXPECTATIONS

"I've failed over and over and over again in my life and that's why I succeed. There is no such thing as a perfect basketball player." -Michael Jordan, NBA player

Unrealistic beliefs and expectations cause emotional pain. Your perception of an experience affects your emotions. Perception is a way of regarding or understanding something. Perfectionism is unrealistic thinking and one of the main causes of stress and fear of failure.

Unrealistic expectations can also cause excessive feelings of disappointment and frustration. An expectation is something looked forward to as likely to occur. If you want and expect life to be easy, you will create unnecessary painful feelings when it doesn't happen. Problems and pain are a part of life.

The belief that people are either winners or losers is unrealistic. Everyone wins and loses, but those experiences don't make us winners or losers. It's better to try and then lose, than to lose by not trying.

We all have successes and failures, but those experiences don't make us a success or a failure. Human beings are imperfect creatures, who must learn by trial and error.

"Even a mistake may turn out to be the
one thing necessary to a worthwhile achievement."
-Henry Ford

Major league baseball players don't expect to get on base every time, but they do expect to get a hit the next time they are up to bat. If they expected to get on base 100% of the time they would feel like failures and have little self-confidence. They must accept the reality that it's hard to get on base and batting .300 is very good.

"Every strike brings me closer to the next home run."
-Babe Ruth

Professional bull riders face real danger and emotional ups and downs. To be a successful bull rider you must believe in yourself and control your imagination. Bull riders block out many traumatic experiences and visualize successful rides. They must focus on the present moment to perform well. Riding rank bulls is difficult and if you ride 50% of the bulls you get on, you are doing well. Successful bull riders must have realistic expectations and believe they can ride the next bull they are getting on.

To cope with the challenges of life, you can adopt the belief that losing and winning doesn't make you a loser or a winner. You can learn to use positive suggestions and mental pictures to achieve goals and create the emotions you want. You can be successful, but you can never be perfect.

"I have not failed. I've just found 10,000
ways that won't work." -Thomas Edison

Donnie Osmond has been performing on stage since he was five years old. He gradually developed stage fright. He became so nervous before going on stage, he almost retired from the entertainment business. His wife cured his stage fright by helping Donnie to realize he was trying to be perfect.

As soon as Donnie realized the tremendous pressure he created by his unrealistic expectations, he was free to enjoy entertaining people again.

Perfectionism defeats many people. Many people give up trying new things or commit suicide because of their mistakes. A more realistic and relaxed attitude will help you deal with whatever challenges you face.

When parents have unrealistic expectations for their child, they create stress and frustration for themselves and their child. Children often see their parents as god-like creatures until they grow up. Then some adults blame their parents for past mistakes, as if their parents should be perfect. Children and parents need to have realistic expectations if they want to create better relationships.

Married couples often expect too much of their mates. Everyone is imperfect and have good and bad personality traits. If we focus on their flaws and ignore the good qualities, we aren't seeing the whole person. Realistic expectations are essential for relationships and coping with life.

People are not winners or losers. Winners and losers are temporary labels given to people and their behaviors. We are spirit beings in temporary bodies.

"We are all full of weakness and errors; let us mutually pardon each other our follies." -Voltaire

EMOTIONAL PAIN

It's a myth that people carry pain from a past experience in their subconscious mind. If it was possible to carry pain, then it would also be possible to carry pleasure.

Our brains and nervous systems create emotions depending on what we are experiencing or imagining. Pleasant feelings can be created as quickly as painful feelings.

Someone reliving a past experience is actually replaying memories using their imagination. Replaying painful memories causes the brain and nervous system to create many of the same feelings that were felt in the past.

146

Memories are imaginary and have no real power over us. We aren't ruined because of past mistakes or traumatic experiences, even if we believe we are. Everyone experiences painful and pleasurable moments and those memories are stored in the brain. Stop giving power to the past by focusing on the present moment and controlling your imagination.

Dealing with pain is one the toughest things we have to do. When you are hurt by another person, it's important to learn from the experience and become a wiser person. One of the worst things to do is become bitter and hold a grudge.

We all learn by trial and error. No one is ever ruined by a painful experience. Look for the lesson to be learned in each experience. Life is a learning process with painful and pleasurable experiences.

STAGES OF GRIEF

The definition of grief is deep sorrow, caused by loss or someone's death. Elisabeth Kubler-Ross wrote a book called *On Death and Dying.*

In her book she writes about the five stages of grief which she believes are denial, anger, bargaining, depression and acceptance. Her theory has been accepted by many people, but has not been proven.

I know a woman named Mary who watched her husband kill himself with a gun. She went to see a counselor, who told her she needed to go through the five stages of grief.

The counselor told Mary she was in denial and needed to realize her husband was dead. Mary said, "You don't know what you're talking about. I'm not in denial. I was there when my husband killed himself." Mary had already accepted her husband was dead and wasn't in denial.

147

When my sister died in a boating accident, I didn't know how to cope with the loss. I was 25 years old and had never been through something that painful before. I didn't go through a denial or bargaining stage, but I did experience anger and depression.

When my father died from a heart attack, I didn't become angry, deny he was dead or bargain with God. Each person deals with a loss in their own way depending on their beliefs and perception of the event. Painful feelings are a common part of loss, but denial, anger or bargaining sometimes are not.

Feelings of sorrow or happiness are created by words and images. It's impossible to miss someone if you don't think about the person.

To overcome feelings of sorrow, you can stop creating them and change how you perceive each loss. When you remember the person, choose to remember the good times and then when you think about the person you will feel better. If you died, would you want those who love you to be sad?

"The most beautiful people we have known are those who have known defeat, known suffering, known struggle, known loss, and have found their way out of those depths."
-Elisabeth Kubler-Ross

"Remember me with smiles and laughter, for that's the way I'll remember you all. If you can only remember me with tears, then don't remember me at all."
- Michael Landon (Eugene Orowitz)

"Never forget the three powerful resources you always have available to you: love, prayer, and forgiveness."
-H. Jackson Brown, Jr.

EMOTIONS AND BELIEFS

Emotions are strong feelings. Feelings are electrical and chemical reactions in the body. It is a misconception that feelings are beliefs. When we visualize a possible experience in the future, we create feelings. The words, images and feelings create a belief and an expectation of possible success or failure.

When we think positive we are using positive words and images to create feelings, beliefs and expectations. Confidence is the belief in one's ability to succeed. Our past experiences and knowledge affect our current beliefs, expectations and confidence. Words and imagery can create hope or despair.

FORGIVENESS AND GUILT

The definition of forgive is cancel a debt, stop feeling angry or resentful toward someone for an offense, flaw, or mistake. If you want to be happier you must learn to forgive yourself and others for their mistakes and selfishness. Forgiveness helps us let go of the past and move on.

Everyone has past traumatic experiences. Visualizing the painful memories over and over only reinforces them.

The definition of guilt is the fact of having committed an offense or crime. Guilt is also a feeling caused by believing you have done something bad or wrong. Many times we feel guilty and punish ourselves for the mistakes we made which were unavoidable. The word sin means an offense or mistake. Mistakes are a necessary part of the learning and growing process.

149

Human beings are controlled by beliefs and some of their beliefs create unrealistic expectations and guilt. Many parents feel guilt because of unavoidable mistakes they made while raising their children. People often seek to stop painful feelings of guilt by self-punishment, drugs, seeing priests or psychiatrists.

Many combat soldiers suffer from post traumatic stress disorder because they are overwhelmed by feelings of guilt and they don't control their imaginations. The military trains men to kill, but drill instructors don't teach them how to cope with guilt which can come from killing.

Grudges cause pain when we think of the person or experience. The definition of a grudge is a persistent feeling of resentment towards someone. It's far better to forgive the person and stop believing you are ruined by past experiences.

Holding grudges and replaying painful experiences over and over is like carrying a big heavy suitcase. It's a good idea to unpack the painful memories and travel light through life with a carry-on bag filled with many pleasant memories. You can then pull them out and look at them when you want to feel good.

WORRY

"Our doubts are traitors because they make us lose the good we might win by fearing to attempt." -William Shakespeare

One definition of the word worry is to have a troubled mind. Worry is a state of anxiety and uncertainty over actual or potential problems. Worry is created when we visualize unpleasant experiences from our past or painful experiences in our future.

150

The mental pictures may seem real to us. The brain and nervous system create proper emotions as if they are reality. We may then react as if they are reality. Reality is how things truly are, regardless of our beliefs and perceptions. Reality is how things actually exist, rather than as they may appear or might be imagined. When we let our imagination run wild, we are not fully reacting to the present moment. Post Traumatic Stress Disorder is a good example of worry.

We cannot create our own world by visualizing it. Mental hospitals are full of people who perceive the world in their own way. Every culture and religion creates beliefs which affect perceptions. Reality is what it is, regardless of all the myths and lies we learn.

When we take control of our imagination and self-talk, we can stop 90% of the fear and pain we will suffer in life. Focusing on the present moment and working on a worthwhile goal is a good remedy for worry.

Worry can be a positive process if used temporarily to avoid making the same mistakes. Painful experiences can teach great lessons and be used to achieve goals.

Experience and knowledge are needed to achieve whatever goals we desire. The past is gone and the memories have no power to hurt us, unless we replay them.

Prayer is a great way to focus our attention. Prayer can be a very powerful way to use words and images. When we visualize a positive outcome, then positive feelings will be created

Positive thinking is using words and images in a realistic and productive way. Learning to relax and control your thoughts will make your life better.

FEAR

Fear is an electrical and chemical reaction in the body. Fear is another word for anxiety, tension, nervousness or excitement. You will not create fear if you remain physically relaxed.

Fear is created by real or imagined danger. The word danger means a person or thing that is likely to cause harm or injury. Fear is the nervousness which comes when we encounter or imagine something dangerous.

Fear is not like a tiger that attacks. Franklin Delano Roosevelt said, "We have nothing to fear but fear itself." He may not have understood what fear actually is.

When we face our fears and overcome them, we are actually learning how to stay more relaxed by controlling our words and imagery.

When you become nervous, it doesn't mean you are a coward. Getting butterflies before performing can help you perform better.

Nervous feelings are caused by your body getting ready to react to something which may be dangerous and cause pain.

The fear factor is actually the pain factor. Mental toughness is the ability to face and endure pain. It's also the ability to ignore pain.

Some people don't have a high pain threshold. They are motivated more by the desire to avoid pain than the desire to have pleasure. Most people seek pleasure in safe ways, but some people love dangerous activities.

Fear can be pleasurable or painful. Some people love the adrenaline rush from watching a horror movie. They may not realize the music, words and imagery cause the excitement called fear. There are people who go on roller coasters to create the pleasurable rush of hormones.

Adrenaline is a powerful hormone which can help you perform better if it is controlled. It can also cause you to freeze up or choke when there is too much released into the bloodstream. When you keep your muscles relaxed, focus on the present moment and control your words and imagery, you will not create as much fear.

COURAGE

The definition of the word courage is the ability to confront fear, danger and painful experiences.

Courage is controlling the imagination and acting in spite of danger and possible pain. Without courage we cannot face life aggressively and overcome the obstacles needed to create a better life.

Courage is deciding to go after what you desire regardless of the pain you may experience. Without real or imagined danger, the feeling of fear isn't created. Having courage is a choice.

PHOBIAS

The word phobia is another word for fear. The brain naturally creates anxiety as a reaction to real or imagined danger. Anxiety isn't a disease or a mental disorder.

The cure for most anxiety is to control your thinking and train your brain to react the way you want. Anxiety attacks can also be caused by diet, drugs or demons.

When a person says they have the fear of flying, they are actually afraid of the plane not flying. They visualize the plane crashing and being hurt or killed. The mental pictures create anxiety and the desire to avoid getting on a plane.

153

Most people can drive down a busy freeway 70 mph and remain calm, because they don't visualize getting in an accident.

When fear is caused by snakes, the response is usually triggered when there is a snake present. When anxiety is created by germs it can become an almost continuous state of tension, because we cannot see germs and they are everywhere.

A germ phobia can become an obsessive compulsive habit. With practice the mental pictures become more vivid and the emotional state is created almost instantly. Images of becoming ill often trigger compulsive cleaning.

Exposure to what makes you nervous can help to desensitize you to it, provided you don't get hurt doing it. Many phobias are caused by past experiences or by what we were taught.

A friend of mine had a fear of lightning and thunder. Her friends thought she was being irrational and told her it was all in her mind. Jamey's fear started as a little girl, when lightning struck her house. From that moment on, she automatically reacted with life or death emotions during a thunderstorm. She wasn't controlling her imagination.

She was reacting as if the experience was happening again because of her mental pictures. I helped Jamey overcome her phobia by using a simple technique which will work with most phobias.

I taught Jamey to control her emotions by controlling her words and imagery. I also taught her how to train her brain. Each day she created new memories in which she was safe. She also rehearsed a new way to automatically react.

At the end of the three weeks she no longer reacted to a thunderstorm as if it was a life or death experience.

PHOBIA REMOVAL EXERCISE

1. Do the relaxation exercise to become focused and relaxed.
2. Visualize yourself going through the experience safely.
3. Use positive self-talk.
4. Practice this exercise daily for a minimum of three weeks. It usually takes time and practice to create new automatic responses and habits.

First, Jamey did the relaxation exercise to relax her muscles and focus her attention on one thing.

Second, she visualized herself in a thunderstorm. She created vivid mental pictures, until she became nervous. Her brain and nervous system reacted as if there was real danger.

Third, she said to herself, "You are safe. The lightning and thunder aren't going to hurt you. Relax. Take a deep breath and relax. What happened to you years ago isn't going to happen now."

Fourth, she calmed herself down and then opened her eyes.

Fifth, Jamey practiced this technique two times a day for three weeks. Each time she mentally rehearsed being in a thunderstorm her brain recorded the experience as if it was a real experience.

This form of mental rehearsal can be used to overcome other fears, such as the fear of flying. The key to success is visualizing yourself flying on the plane and landing safely over and over again.

The more vivid the mental pictures are the faster your brain and nervous system will react and create emotions. Each imagined safe flight will be recorded as a memory and gradually create the belief you will not be hurt if you fly.

155

SELF-CONTROL TIPS

Keeping busy helps break the worry habit. Focus on what you are doing in the present moment. It's hard to be depressed or worry when you're busy having fun or working on a challenging project.

Practice keeping your muscles more relaxed as you work, play and live your life. Think of yourself as a marathon runner instead of a sprinter. If you try to hurry and go fast all day long, you will be exhausted at the end of the day. Breathing and moving slower will help you maintain a more relaxed attitude.

Stop watching television and listening to the radio when you want to relax. They both stimulate your brain.

Accept the fact that everyone is imperfect. Develop realistic expectations. Strive to improve, but never expect perfection. Perfectionism can keep your self-esteem and self-confidence low.

When competing and in everyday life, focus on doing your best, not comparing yourself to others.

Use a relaxation break whenever you can. Even five minutes of slow breathing or walking can help to release tension in your muscles. Use your trigger word relax to help you create the feeling of relaxation.

Take time for a nap if possible.

Become your own best friend. Stop beating yourself up with negative words and images. Take the time to say positive affirmations and visualize pleasant memories.

Believe in mental telepathy and develop faith in yourself and God. Prayer can help you live with more courage and confidence. Prayer is a form of positive thinking.

Stretching and exercise are great for releasing tension. When you become tense, sometimes all you need is to change your focus, move around and take a few slow deep breaths.

"What do you do with a mistake: recognize it, learn from it, forget it." -Dean Smith, U.S. Olympic coach

SUMMARY

1. Relaxation is a lack of muscle tension.
2. Emotions are electrical and chemical reactions to stimuli such as sounds, words and images.
3. You can control your emotions when you control what you focus your attention on.
4. Think of the word wit as an acronym for Word Imagery Thinking. Your brain operates using words and images.
5. Use the CAN technique to control your emotions. CAN is an acronym for Change Attention Now. When you refocus your attention, your emotions will change.
6. People are usually controlled by their beliefs and feelings. Your desire to feel pleasure, or avoid pain, are controlling a lot of your choices and behavior.
7. To achieve any goal you must be willing to suffer some pain. 90% of the pain we feel in life is created by our own words and images.
8. Forgive yourself and others for their mistakes, so you can move on. Stop replaying traumatic memories.
9. Fear is another word for anxiety, tension or excitement. You can control fear and worry when you take control of your imagination.
10. When you practice the relaxation exercise and the CAN technique everyday, you will develop more self-control.
11. Start taking action to control your emotions.

*"He has achieved success
who has lived well,
laughed often and loved much;
who has gained the respect
of intelligent men and
the love of little children;
who has left the world
better than he found it."*

-Bessie A. Stanley

CHAPTER ELEVEN

Addiction Secrets

*"Our greatest glory is not in never failing,
but in rising up every time we fail."*
- Ralph Waldo Emerson

As you read this chapter, you will be empowering yourself with knowledge and developing a greater understanding of addiction, chemical dependency and recovery. You will discover how to escape the pleasure and pain trap.

There are two types of habitual behaviors; healthy and unhealthy habits. A habit is something done often, easily and without much thought.

The brain is a habit machine. Over 90 percent of our feelings and actions are habitual. It takes practice before our brains are trained to do things automatically. It usually takes approximately 21 days to create a new habit or let go of an old one.

The saying, "use it or lose it," applies to habits as well as muscles. Ivan Pavlov trained his dogs to salivate when they heard the sound of a bell. He would ring the bell before he fed them. After enough repetitions, the dogs eventually associated the bell with food. The dogs responded automatically without conscious thought. The desire for food was triggered by the bell.

When Pavlov wanted to stop the auto-response, he stopped bringing the food after ringing the bell. Gradually, the dogs no longer associated the bell with food. Habits are thinking, feeling and acting patterns that must be reinforced to remain strong.

Some learned habits are called obsessive compulsive disorders. A compulsion is a desire to do something. An OCD is characterized by obsessive thinking, cravings and repetitive behaviors. The word aholic means, someone who is obsessed with something.

ADDICTIONS ARE HABITS

A habit is sometimes called an addiction when the person wants to stop the behavior, but finds it difficult to do so. The definition of the word addict is someone who has *surrendered* to a strong habit. Everyone has strong habits.

Addictions can be healthy or unhealthy. Unhealthy habits can involve many things, such as drugs, cussing, food, gambling, cellphones, video games, sex, germs, exercising, sports, money, shopping, worrying, or lying. Many people love their obsessive behaviors and don't perceive them as unhealthy or strong habits until they try to stop.

Everyone has addictions and we're all addicts. We all have addictive personalities, because we are creatures of habit.

ADDICTIONS AREN'T DISEASES

An addiction is a habit, not an incurable disease. Some habitual behaviors, such as drinking alcohol do cause physical disease symptoms, because alcohol is a poison.

Will power is sometimes misunderstood. The definition of the word will is the power of making a reasoned choice, or of controlling one's own actions. Will, also means to desire, crave or want.

Your will power is usually controlled by habitual thinking patterns and beliefs. Most people believe they are making reasoned choices and using will power when they are actually responding automatically like Pavlov's dogs.

Cravings are desires. Desire is a strong feeling of wanting something. Cravings are often automatic responses triggered by words or images.

Many people who habitually use drugs have surrendered their choices and desires to demons. Demons can train human beings to want drugs. They can make them believe they are *powerless* and can't control themselves. Many addicts believe they can't or don't want to live without their drug. It's those beliefs which trap them.

In the country of India, people train elephants to work. Training starts when the elephant is first taken from its mother. The trainer ties the small elephant to a sturdy post with a strong chain.

The small elephant will pull against the chain until it's convinced it cannot break free. Later when the elephant is big enough to break a strong chain, it won't try. The elephant can then be tied up with a small rope, because it believes it's powerless and can't break free.

If you stop using a drug, but still want to use it, you will create mental pain. As long as a person is in a love and hate relationship with a chemical, there will be a tug of war.

Addictions are habits, not physical diseases. Some habits are healthy and others are unhealthy. Everyone seeks ways to feel happy. Using drugs is just one way people habitually seek to feel good.

ACTIVITY ADDICTIONS

There are two types of chemical addictions. Human beings use activities and poisons to alter their feelings. Both types of behavior involve hormones the body produces.

Some people love to gamble or watch sports, because these behaviors cause the brain to release adrenaline and other hormones. Our own chemicals can be very addictive, because they give us the feeling everyone wants. This feeling is pleasure or happiness.

The problem with many activities is they can also cause pain if not controlled. Shopaholics spend too much money. Gamblers lose too much money and sex addicts ruin relationships or their health. People can become ill from over exercising or working too much.

Attention addiction is common and some people crave the constant attention and approval of other people. When two people fall in love, they get "high" on hormones. If the relationship ends, they will miss the pleasurable feelings.

When the pleasure people get from activities or drugs stops being worth the pain, it's called hitting rock bottom. Rock bottom is different for each person. Some people have higher pain thresholds than other people. Pain and pleasure are great motivators.

A documentary called, *Scared Straight,* showed how fear of prison can help to motivate teenagers to want to stay out of prison. Most people make decisions based on pain and pleasure.

Many activities are fun, dangerous, destructive and addictive. When you repeat a behavior over and over it can become a habitual way of creating pleasurable feelings. The first type of addiction involves activities and hormones our bodies naturally create.

POISON ADDICTIONS

The second type of chemical addiction involves ingesting poisons. This type of addiction can lead to chemical dependency and physical disease. Caffeine, table sugar, cocaine, methadone, heroin, marijuana, alcohol and other poisons stimulate the brain to release adrenaline and other hormones.

These chemicals create pleasure and pain in the body. The pleasurable "high" comes from the poisons and our own hormones. The "low" is the painful symptoms caused from being poisoned. To stop the pain many people use the poison again. People hooked on a drug are chasing the "high".

Poisons create blood sugar and oxygen imbalances which affect energy level and cause feelings of depression. Tobacco, coffee, sodas, alcoholic drinks and other drugs can create a *vicious cycle* called chemical dependency. Seeking energy and pleasure while trying to avoid pain is a trap. Users fall in love with the feelings the poisons create and often ignore the health risks.

When a person loves to drink alcohol, they will do it whether they are happy or sad. This person has found a way to feel good for the moment and release tension.

Alcohol is often used as a crutch or a quick fix for a blood sugar imbalance caused by diet. Many alcoholics suffer from hypoglycemia caused by excess sugar and alcohol.

Comfort foods and drugs are often part of the energy and pleasure seeking trap. Why don't most people reach for fruits and vegetables when they are feeling depressed? Because they don't contain mood altering substances like refined sugar, caffeine, or alcohol. People want to be stimulated or relaxed and usually seek instant gratification.

163

Tobacco users become dependent on the chemicals in tobacco. As the poisons begins to leave the brain, there are withdrawal symptoms. There is also a change in the sugar and oxygen in their bloodstream.

Withdrawal symptoms are anxiety, headache, fatigue, and difficulty concentrating. Because people want to feel good, they use the substance again. They usually love or need the poisons which has enslaved them.

Awareness and knowledge are the keys to escaping the pleasure and pain trap. A person must first want to stop and then associate pain and fear with using the substance.

Some people need intervention because drugs like alcohol, methamphetamine, heroin and many prescription drugs can destroy their ability to think rationally. Their brains are too poisoned to realize the danger they are in and they can't rescue themselves.

"A man takes a drink, the drink takes a drink,
the drink takes the man." -Irish Proverb

Most people who use drugs habitually, don't consciously choose to become trapped. The drugs create a vicious cycle of pleasure, pain and *confusion*. Drug addicts have a lot of will power. They will do almost anything to get that pleasurable feeling again.

Ivan Pavlov trained his dogs to salivate when they heard the sound of a bell. Through repetition the response became a habit. The dogs were trained to associate the pleasurable food with the sound of the bell.

Human beings can be trained like Pavlov's dogs to get excited over things that give them pleasure even if they are unhealthy. Many addicts *surrender* to the poisons they crave.

People crave things which cause pleasure. If you don't get pleasure from gambling or alcohol, you probably won't get hooked on either one. If sex is boring or painful, you probably don't want to have sex. Most chemical addictions are created by habitual pleasure seeking.

FOOD ADDICTIONS

Many of the foods that give us pleasure contain poisons which cause the brain to release hormones. Some people call junk foods, comfort foods. Comfort foods can create pleasurable and painful feelings. They stimulate our taste buds and change our brain chemistry. Millions of Americans love and want addictive substances such as refined sugar, caffeine and alcohol.

Visualizing a food can create a desire to experience the pleasure again. If you want to stop craving certain foods, stop focusing your attention on them. You will need to decide whether the pleasure you temporarily receive is worth the pain, it also creates.

Your beliefs will control your desires. When you believe and expect something is going to be painful, you will usually want to avoid it.

MONKEY TRAPS

"Monkey Trap: a cage containing a banana with a hole large enough for a monkey's hand to fit in, but not large enough for a monkey's fist (clutching the banana) to come out." - Wiktionary

165

A monkey trap is successful when the monkey is *unaware* it can let go of the banana and then escape. Addictions work the same way as a monkey trap. As long as we are unaware that we can let go of our habitual thinking and behaviors, we remain trapped.

The saying, "monkey see, monkey do," applies to people. We all learn by imitating others. Many times we do what other people do without accurate knowledge or concern about the consequences of our actions.

Television, magazines, songs and movies influence our thinking. Advertising agencies are tempting and training us to do many things which are destructive.

ADDICTION RECOVERY BUSINESS

Addiction recovery treatment is a $300 billion per year industry in the U.S. There are over 14,000 drug addiction facilities and fees can be over $60,000. Their success rates are low and relapses are good for the rehab business.

Most recovery programs use the outdated 1930s Alcoholics Anonymous 12 step program. A.A. principles are like a monkey trap because they are *misleading* people and keeping them trapped. The Big Book says you can't let go of your bad habit, because once you become an alcoholic, you'll always be an alcoholic.

" Once an alcoholic, always an alcoholic."
-Alcoholics Anonymous, Big Book

The steps convince people that alcoholism is caused by defects of character, which make them powerless over alcohol. **They ignore the fact that alcohol poisoning is what causes the insane behavior and physical disease.**

166

THE 12 STEPS OF ALCOHOLICS ANONYMOUS

Step 1. We admitted we were **powerless** over alcohol and our lives had become unmanageable.

Step 2. We came to believe that a power greater than ourselves could restore us to **sanity**.

Step 3. We made a decision to turn our will and our lives over to the care of God, as we understand him.

Step 4. We made a searching and fearless moral inventory of ourselves.

Step 5. We admitted to God, to ourselves, and to another human being the exact nature of our wrongs.

Step 6. We were entirely ready to have God remove all these **defects of character.**

Step 7. We humbly asked him to remove our shortcomings.

Step 8. We made a list of all persons we had harmed, and became willing to make amends to them all.

Step 9. We made direct amends to such people, whenever possible, except when to do so would injure them or others.

Step 10. We continued to take personal inventory, and when we were wrong, promptly admitted it.

Step 11. We sought through prayer and meditation to improve our conscious contact with God, as we understand him, praying only for knowledge of his will and the power to carry that out.

Step 12. Having had a spiritual awakening as the result of these steps, we tried to carry this message to others, and practice these principles in all of our affairs.

METHADONE TREATMENT

Methadone treatment is a good example of how some doctors are misleading their patients. They substitute heroin for another harmful drug. Methadone is a highly addictive poison which causes suicide, chemical dependency, disease and death.

HOW TO BECOME AN ALCOHOLIC

Start drinking beverages which contain the mind-altering drug called alcohol. When you are drinking, you will become more irrational with each drink. The reasoning part of the brain will be impaired.

Next, drink alcohol every day. One glass of wine or a beer is enough to start. You will create a habitual desire for alcohol if you like the feelings it creates. You will also start creating chemical dependency.

Now, drink more alcohol each day so your body will develop tolerance to the poison and the desire for it will increase. Your irrational thinking and behavior will also increase. You will probably develop a blood sugar disorder called hypoglycemia and become chemically dependent.

At this point it will seem normal to be intoxicated every day. You will probably want and need alcohol to feel good. You will not perceive how irrational you are. Your brain is now under the influence of alcohol 24 hours a day. You aren't in denial. You are unable to realize how poisoned and damaged your brain has become.

Congratulations, you are now an alcoholic with chronic alcoholism. You are in a pleasure and pain trap.

ALCOHOL POISONING

"Experience shows that when an alcoholic succeeds in getting off alcohol, he usually substitutes sweets. This is because almost all alcoholics are hypoglycemic, and sugar provides the same temporary lift that alcohol once did."
-Dr. Robert C. Atkins

Alcohol is a poison excreted by yeast. It's a colorless, volatile, pungent liquid, in fermented liquors. Alcoholic drinks also contain concentrated sugar.

An alcoholic is someone suffering from alcohol poisoning and a blood sugar imbalance. Irrational behavior, physical illness and chemical dependency are the results of habitually drinking beverages which contain alcohol.

Alcohol and other drugs are acidic. Green juice therapy helps drug users detox in a less painful way. Fruits and vegetables alkalize the body and supply nutrients which the body needs to heal.

"I am more afraid of alcohol than of all the bullets of the enemy."
-Stonewall Jackson,
U.S. Civil War general

SHE QUIT LOVING BOOZE THAT DAY

Once a drunk, always a drunk.
That's what she learned at A.A.
She believed all of their myths,
until she passed away.
She was taught at the meetings,
don't blame alcohol.
Addiction is a disease,
and it's not your choice at all.
One day at a time,
the poor misguided soul,
said, "I'm an alcoholic"
and then she played that role.
She fell in love with a drug,
that brings pleasure and pain.
Alcohol is a poison,
that makes people go insane.
When she passed away,
she quit loving wine and beer.
She left her mortal body.
I hope she left her pain and fear.
She quit loving booze that day.
Her body slowly went cold.
Evil spirits went away.
She quit loving booze that day.
They had labeled her a drunk,
but I knew it wasn't true.
We're all creatures of habit,
and addictions are habits too.

ALCOHOLICS ANONYMOUS

"Definition of an alcoholic is an egomaniac with an inferiority complex." -Alcoholics Anonymous, Big Book

The founders of A.A. believed an alcoholic is an egomaniac with an inferiority complex. The Webster's dictionary defines an alcoholic as someone who habitually drinks alcohol liquor excessively, and has chronic alcoholism. To become and remain an alcoholic you *must* habitually drink alcohol excessively.

Many A.A. members believe drinking alcohol is safe for other people, but not them. They ignore the fact that alcohol is a poison excreted by yeast, which causes insanity, pain, disease and death.

"Men and women drink essentially because they like the effect produced by alcohol." -Alcoholics Anonymous

Some members envy people who they believe can drink alcohol normally, and they want to drink again. They *love and fear* the effects produced by alcohol.

Drinking alcohol is the only cause of alcoholism. Alcoholism isn't caused by genetics, low self-esteem, defects of character or allergies. Alcoholism is a physical disease caused by alcohol poisoning.

Alcoholics Anonymous often creates codependency and shame. Many members believe they must go to meetings, share their experiences with others, or they will relapse. They live in fear...one day at a time. Some members are ashamed of themselves and believe they are their past behavior. They don't learn the truth about addiction and alcoholism.

171

A.A. members are often taught addiction and alcoholism are incurable diseases and complete recovery is impossible. They call themselves recovering alcoholics or dry drunks for the rest of their lives. Members reinforce their obsession with alcohol at each meeting.

Most members say, "I'm an alcoholic" at each meeting. Repetition of that affirmation reinforces that belief. Would it help someone change if they said, "I'm a loser" everyday? Would it be helpful to believe once a loser, always a loser?

A.A. support groups are mostly made up of well-meaning people searching for help. Some people who go to meetings are court ordered to attend. The meetings don't involve professional guidance or learning self-control skills.

The 12 step program is unnecessary. You don't need to go to meetings and conform to their principles before you can let go of a bad habit. You can pray to God and get the support of other people without going to A.A.

"The A.A. member has to conform to the principles of recovery. His life actually depends upon obedience to spiritual principles. If he deviates too far, the penalty is sure and swift; he sickens and dies." -Alcoholics Anonymous

A.A. IS A RELIGION

A.A. is an organized religion, which originated from the Oxford Group, soon after Prohibition ended in the 1930s. The religion includes spiritual principles, traditions, prayer and turning your will and life over to God. A.A. meetings are religious services which often include the Lord's Prayer and Serenity Prayer.

"In 1938, friends of John D. Rockefeller Jr. became board members." -Alcoholics Anonymous, The birth of A.A.

Bill Wilson, a Wall Street stockbroker and many rich and powerful men promoted this religious organization. **A.A. believes alcohol is harmless if you can drink it normally.**

NORMAL DRINKING

"Many people can drink normally and suffer no physical, mental or social ill effects." - A.A.

Normal drinking without ill effects is a myth. Everyone who drinks alcohol is affected in negative ways. If alcohol is harmless then why would it be illegal to drink until you are 21?

Loss of control, accidents, hangovers, vomiting, violence, unwanted pregnancies, birth defects, suicides, insanity and death are all part of the alcohol experience.

There are approximately 100,000 alcohol related deaths each year in the United States. According to the National Institute on Alcohol Abuse and Alcoholism, approximately 1,800 college students die each year from alcohol-related injuries. Alcohol kills more teenagers than all illegal drugs combined.

The Institute also says over 700,000 college students are assaulted by other students who are under the influence of alcohol. Approximately 599,000 college students are unintentionally injured while intoxicated. Some college students overdose and die because of alcohol binge drinking.

"About six times everyday someone in the United States
dies of alcohol poisoning after drinking too much
in a single binge." -Kim Painter, USA TODAY

Alcohol companies want us to believe drinking alcohol is harmless and fun. Wineries promote images of romance and fine living to their brand of poison. U.S. alcohol sales total over $400 billion per year.

Wine drinkers love the feelings created by alcohol. Does it make sense to believe one glass of wine is healthy, but more is unhealthy? If one glass of wine is healthy and harmless why not give it to small children and pregnant women?

TOBACCO POISONING

Tobacco companies also want us to believe smoking is harmless. Today, millions of people realize cigarettes contain unhealthy and addictive substances. In the 1960s the AMA and many doctors endorsed smoking and told their patients smoking is harmless as long as you don't smoke excessively.

If we use the same logic with tobacco as A.A. uses for alcohol, we will become confused. We'll believe tobacco is harmless if you smoke normally, and the tobacco user's defects of character, low self-esteem, addictive personality, allergies or genetics are the problem.

We'll be wondering why can't everyone smoke cigarettes *normally*. Tobacco is harmless isn't it? Some smokers are unable to use tobacco in moderation and responsibly. They don't know when to say when.

Alcoholism is defined as the habitual excessive drinking of alcohol liquor, and a resulting disease condition. Tobaccoism is the habitual excessive use of tobacco, and a resulting disease condition. Both diseases are caused by poisons. If we believe tobacco is harmless, then tobaccoism would be seen as an insidious disease, like alcoholism. The excessive smoker would be viewed as someone who has lost control and has two diseases. One disease is tobaccoism and the other is addiction.

Why aren't ex-smokers called recovering smokers? Why are ex-alcohol drinkers labeled alcoholics for the rest of their lives? Both are bad habits which involve using poisonous substances which cause chemical dependency and disease.

Many addiction recovery beliefs are unrealistic. Good and bad habits can be started, stopped and then started again. Habits are like clothes that can be changed.

HEROIN POISONING

Imagine being told heroin is harmless as long as you use it *normally.* You are told to use heroin responsibly, or in moderation. If you can't control yourself, you are labeled an addict and told you need a 12 step program.

Group therapy may convince you that heroin didn't cause your addiction. You may be told addiction is a disease and you suffer from an addictive personality and defects of character.

Is this logical thinking? Heroin is a powerful mind-altering drug that can take away our ability to make reasoned choices and cause chemical dependency.

175

WORKAHOLIC

Imagine you are labeled a workaholic and told you will always be a workaholic. You are ill, because you work excessively instead of *normally.* If you use the same logic as the 12 steps of A.A. you will become confused and trapped.

You may think you have an incurable disease called workism and the only hope for you is meetings and total *abstinance* from work. You must live one day at a time, for the rest of your life, as a recovering workaholic.

If you go to 12 step meetings you'll learn to say, "Hi, I'm a workaholic," over and over until you believe it. The other members may convince you the meetings are your only hope. By sharing your personal stories with others, you will help yourself and others to stop working and remain unemployed.

Members of A.A. will tell you, "the steps work...if you work the steps!" The problem is you can't work the steps because they require work and cause relapse.

Does this kind of thinking make sense?
Addictions are strong habits, not incurable diseases.

CHOICES

Some of our behaviors are healthy and some are unhealthy. It's up to each one of us to decide what we want most in our lives.

Relapses are choices. They can be caused by wanting to continue the behavior or the gradual letting go of a strong habit. It took days for Ivan Pavlov to condition his dogs to associate food with the sound of a bell and automatically salivate. It also took days to stop that automatic response. The conditioning usually takes over 21 days of reinforcement.

You can decide to train your brain to have new beliefs and habits, or you can continue the old ones. Only you can decide what's most important to you. What do you desire the most?

SELECTIVE MEMORIES

People usually create mental pictures before making choices. We replay memories or create new images. We associate pain or pleasure to each one.

Before deciding what to eat, we visualize what would taste good. It is the images we create that will affect our choices. People usually avoid restaurants where they have gotten food poisoning, because of the bad memories.

When someone drinks too much and then vomits, that person may say, "I'll never drink again." The same person may later ignore the painful memory and visualize a pleasurable drinking experience before drinking again. Mental pictures cause a person to believe the future experience will be painful or pleasurable.

HABIT CHANGING EXERCISE

Practice this exercise everyday until you no longer want to repeat the behavior.

Visualize painful experiences caused by your unhealthy habit. With repetition you will eventually associate pain and fear with that behavior and not want to do it anymore.

Next, visualize yourself being happy and healthy no longer doing the behavior. Think about all the benefits you will receive by changing your habit and creating a new one.

Now, tell yourself, I can and will change my behavior. I will create a better life. I will stop reinforcing the unwanted habit and the cravings will eventually fade away.

177

"Anyone can quit a bad habit, but you have to really want to quit. You have to make up your mind."
-Waylon Jennings, Singer

ADDICTION REMOVAL TIPS

1. Make a choice and a commitment. You must really want to stop your bad habit now!
2. Interrupt the automatic response when it's triggered. You can say no, stop, shut up demons, etc. Then focus your attention on something else to stop the cravings.
3. Train your brain to associate pain to the habit by visualizing painful experiences.
4. Change your beliefs about the activity or substance so you lose your desire for it.
5. Tell yourself everyday, the pleasure you get from the behavior isn't worth the pain, it also causes.
6. Visualize yourself being happy without using the activity or substance until you believe you can. Focus on the benefits of changing your behavior.
7. Practice the relaxation exercise and CAN technique everyday. Learn to release stress and take more control of your words and images.
8. Pray to God for strength, guidance and protection from evil spirits.
9. Reach out to friends or family for support. Avoid friends and environments which encourage the bad behavior.
10. Don't give up. Some habits take more time and practice to break.
11. Realize you are not your habits. Good and bad addictions are like clothes that can be changed.

CHAPTER TWELVE

Self-Discovery

"To be yourself in a world that is constantly trying to make you something else is the greatest accomplishment."
-Ralph Waldo Emerson

Self-discovery is the act or process of gaining knowledge and understanding of your abilities, feelings, true potential, character and motives.

THE POWER OF BELIEFS

Changing your beliefs is one major key to changing your life. A belief is an idea you assume to be the truth. It affects your perception of yourself and the world.

Many people are trapped by self-defeating beliefs and habits. They believe they cannot change, because they believe their habits are who they really are. Beliefs and habits are sometimes hard to change even though we know they are wrong or unhealthy.

Fear of pain also stops many people from changing. Some beliefs are like sinking ships. Unless we abandon them, we go down with them.

"To find yourself, think for yourself. The highest form of human excellence is to question oneself and others."
-Socrates

Your personality is mainly a collection of learned and practiced thinking patterns. Beliefs about yourself and the world will influence how you will think, feel and act. A change in beliefs and habits will change your personality.

If you were diagnosed by a group of doctors and told you had an incurable cancer, would you believe them? What if the doctors told you to go home and prepare to die because you had only two to six months to live. Would you believe the doctors? Words create beliefs and have the power to inspire or defeat us.

If you are convinced you are stupid, it will affect your ability to learn. Your parents can greatly affect your perception of yourself and the world. Many of our beliefs, desires and behaviors were not created by us alone. People learn what to believe and how to act.

THE POWER OF EXPECTATIONS

Ty Murray is a co-founder of the Professional Bull Riders. When he was born, his parents took him home from the hospital in a cowboy hat and boots.

Ty was taught that he was a cowboy. The first sentence he spoke was, "I'm a bull rider." When Ty was three years old, he started riding calves.

Ty's parents told him he would break Larry Mahan's record by winning seven all-around titles. He was also told he would become king of the cowboys someday.

Ty expected to achieve those goals, because he believed his parents. He practiced and worked hard to develop the skills needed to accomplish the goals. Eventually, Ty won seven all around titles and fulfilled his parents' dream. His parents used words to influence his desires, beliefs and behavior.

TALENT

The definition of the word talent is a special ability which allows someone to do something well. Successful people know talents and skills are improved by practice. Almost anyone can learn to sing, dance or play a musical instrument if they do the work required. Each person is born with strengths and weaknesses. Talent alone is not enough.

Great athletes, dancers, singers and musicians are created, not born. They must work hard to achieve their goals. To be good at any job requires knowledge and training. Focus on doing your best and you will gradually get better with practice.

A friend of mine is a professional artist. He has taught many children to develop their artistic abilities. Some children have the unrealistic belief that good artists are born, not made. Terry gives children the basic knowledge they need to develop artistic skills and he helps them believe they can become good artists if they practice.

THE POWER OF HYPNOSIS

"If we doubted our fears instead of doubting our dreams, imagine how much we'd accomplish."
-Jim Brown, NFL player

181

Hypnosis is a state of consciousness in which a person is highly focused and responsive to suggestion. Hypnotists control the brain and nervous system of their subjects. While in a trance, people believe and perceive differently. They become puppets or actors of the hypnotist.

The word perception is defined as the ability to see, hear, or become aware of something through the senses. It's also a way of understanding or interpreting something.

When someone is hypnotized they surrender their free will to the hypnotist. Hypnotists use words to create new beliefs and control behavior. Words have the power to create trances and belief spells. Advertisers use words and images to program people to desire their products. Most people are unaware they are being trained like Pavlov's dogs.

When a hypnotized person is convinced the room is hot, the person will start to sweat. If the hypnotist says an onion is an apple the person will perceive it as an apple. The onion will look, smell and taste like an apple.

A hypnotized person can be told to see and hear things that are not real. They can also develop amnesia and the inability to feel pain. These phenomenons are the natural abilities of our computer-like brains.

A hypnotist can control the imagination of their subjects. When totally focused on the present moment, there are no memories being replayed to interfere with present behavior. The hypnotist tells a person what reality is and who they are. The person then acts out that role.

The words can, can't, and need are powerful. If you tell yourself over and over, I can't live without someone or something, you are training yourself to believe it's true. You are programming a belief. Repetition of words is one method used to create beliefs.

Some people believe they need coffee, alcohol and other drugs to be happy, or make it through the day. Their words create and reinforce their beliefs. Words, images and beliefs affect our desires.

BELIEF SYSTEMS

When a person joins the military, they are sent to a base for basic training. The recruits are given dog tags to identify their bodies. While the person is in training, new beliefs and habits are created by drill instructors. The process is done using "well proven" mind control techniques.

When the process is finished, the recruits have been trained to follow orders without using free will. Drill instructors are like hypnotists and animal trainers who create obedient dog-like behaviors.

If the conditioning has been successful, the soldier will torture or kill innocent people when ordered to do so. They may also perceive their behaviors as justified or heroic.

Human beings can be programmed to believe evil is good and good is evil. Beliefs affect our ability to tell right from wrong and what's real from imaginary.

Religions are belief systems. Each group of people believe they have the facts. Faith in any religion requires indoctrination until the follower is convinced the ideas are true. Faith is defined as unquestioning belief.

The sciences are also belief systems. Many scientific theories are presented as if they are proven facts. Faith in any science requires indoctrination until the follower is convinced the ideas are true. The sciences have many unquestioning believers.

183

SELF-IMAGE PSYCHOLOGY

"This self-image is our own conception of the "sort of person I am. It has been built up from our own beliefs about ourselves." -Maxwell Maltz, M.D.

One definition of an image is a mental picture. The self-image which Maxwell Maltz was referring to is made of many mental pictures and beliefs. A self-image is actually a memory which affects what you believe about yourself.

It's mental pictures which create feelings of confidence or insecurity. We must take control of these images if we want to experience more confidence and happiness.

Your personality and identity is shaped by your past experiences and the beliefs that were created. If you develop dementia or amnesia, you can lose your identity. We are playing roles and need memories to know what to believe and how to perform.

CONFORMITY

"All the world's a stage, and all the men and women are merely players." -William Shakespeare

All the world is a stage and all the men, women and children are playing roles. As children, we are taught what to believe and how to act. Most people accept the reality of the world presented to them. They conform to many of the customs of their culture.

Some people conform to the latest fashion. They wear costumes and alter their natural appearances. Each person learns to fit in and measure their self-worth by different standards. We are affected by peer pressure.

184

Masculine and feminine role playing is part of each culture throughout the world. Some men believe smoking cigars and drinking alcohol are masculine behaviors, while many women believe wearing cosmetics is beauty enhancing and feminine behavior.

The entertainment industry manipulates us. We are influenced by sitcoms, commercials, songs, magazines, movies and books which create many of our beliefs and desires. They are selling us ideas and products.

Many people imitate and idolize actors, athletes and other entertainers. Norma Jeane Mortenson (Marilyn Monroe) was turned into a sex symbol. Her image is false and misleading. Airbrushed and computer generated images create unrealistic standards.

Some people seek a sense of identity or self-worth by obtaining college degrees and titles. Other people become obsessed with power, money, fame, or attractive images.

There are high achievers who suffer from feelings of inferiority. Their insecurity is caused by unrealistic beliefs and expectations. Many of them strive for more money and success, because they never feel good enough.

Those who truly love us, don't love us because of our outer appearances or successes. They love us because of who we are on the inside and how we treat them.

LABELS

"I figured that if I said it enough, I would convince the world that I really was the greatest. It's repetition of affirmations that lead to belief." -Muhammad Ali, boxer

185

People often classify each other by their behaviors. A doctor, lawyer, cowboy, janitor, or secretary is not what a person is. They are only jobs that people do.

Sometimes we think of each other as winners, losers, heroes, cowards, sinners or saints. These are labels for people's behaviors.

We are not our past behavior. We can break free of the past when we start living in the present moment and realize we are spirit beings in temporary bodies.

Our behaviors and beliefs are like costumes which can be changed. We are actors on the stage of life. No one is inferior or superior to other people, and no amount of success or failure can change that fact.

BELIEF EXERCISE

"The minute that we change our minds, and stop giving power to the past, the past with its mistakes loses its power over us." -Maxwell Maltz, M.D.

Do you have unrealistic expectations? Do you believe you should be perfect? Do you believe there are perfect people? Do you believe there are normal and abnormal people? Do you believe status symbols or physical appearances are the ways to measure self-worth?

Take at least 1 hour every week to examine a belief that causes negative feelings. Talk to a friend about that belief to see if it's realistic. You will empower each other with new knowledge and understanding. Awareness of the truth can often set us free.

186

If you want to feel confident and happy more often, then accept yourself and others as imperfect. Practice using words and images to create new beliefs, habits and desired emotions. Tell yourself positive affirmations and visualize pleasant memories everyday. Let go of your grudges and forgive yourself and others for their mistakes and selfishness. We are spirit beings with temporary beliefs and behaviors.

THE POWER OF DESIRE AND WORK

"The will to win is not nearly so
important as the will to prepare to win."
-Vince Lombardi, NFL coach

The definition of desire is to long for, crave, want, wish or will something. To accomplish any goal you must know exactly what you want, become determined to have it and then work hard to achieve it.

Donnie Gay won the World Bull Riding Championship eight times. I interviewed him to find out why he was able to accomplish his goals. He told me it was his desire, effort and positive thinking which made the difference.

Donnie said, "You get out of life what you put into it. No pain, no gain. I wanted to be a world champion bull rider and nothing else was going to satisfy me. I wanted to be the world champion more than most bull riders."

"Genius is one percent inspiration...
and ninety nine percent perspiration."
-Thomas Alva Edison

187

Donnie was willing to do the work and suffer the pain to accomplish his dream. He focused on being the best he could be. Donnie trained his brain using positive words and images. He created a burning desire, determination, self-confidence and great expectations.

Billy Mills won a gold medal at the 1964 Olympics in the 10,000 meter run. He knows the importance of desire and hard work to create a better life. The movie *Running Brave* tells the story of Billy growing up on an Indian Reservation in South Dakota and eventually achieving his dream.

You can create a better life if you want it bad enough and are willing to do the work. Start visualizing what you want and tell yourself over and over I can accomplish my goal. Then go work for your dream. Until you have a burning desire to achieve your goal, it's easy to become distracted or quit.

CONFIDENCE FACTOR

"If you put forth the effort, good things will be bestowed upon you. I've always believed if you put in the work, the results will come." -Michael Jordan

We are confident about things we can do well. We shouldn't have confidence when it comes to things we know little about or have little experience with. Everyone has insecurities. It's normal to sometimes feel uncertain and anxious in a dangerous and complex world.

To feel more confident requires skill, knowledge and the belief that you can handle whatever happens. Some anxiety and insecurity is caused by a lack of successful experiences.

To develop confidence requires successful experiences and that takes practice. Mental rehearsal and physical practice can be used to train your brain. To have more confidence you can visualize future and past successes until you create confident feelings.

CONFIDENCE EXERCISE

One of the best ways to create faith in yourself is to read a list of your past successes. It doesn't matter how small the successes were. Taking fifteen minutes a day to imagine past successes will increase your confidence. Visualize each success vividly until you create the feelings of confidence. Positive words and images will help you create the confidence needed to achieve future goals.

GOAL ACHIEVEMENT TIPS

1. Decide exactly what you want to achieve.
2. Acquire the specialized knowledge needed to create a good plan of action. Learn from others who have been successful achieving a similar goal.
3 Create a plan of action and improve it when needed. Have a daily schedule to follow.
4. Set deadlines for the achievement of your goals.
5. Reduce big goals into smaller short term goals.
6. Don't be afraid of mistakes and pain.
7. Do the work it takes to succeed. Work is the ultimate key to success.

*"Failure is simply the opportunity
to begin again, this time more intelligently."*
-Henry Ford

GOAL ACHIEVEMENT EXERCISE

Read your goals out loud at least once a day. As you read each goal, take time to visualize the goal already achieved. Use positive affirmations to create more faith in yourself. Tell yourself, "I can and will achieve this goal."

The brain and nervous system will react to words and vivid images by creating feelings and beliefs. The visions will be recorded as if you have already achieved the goals.

You are training yourself to do what you desire. You are also training your brain to attract knowledge which will help you achieve your goals.

Follow your plan of action and keep your eye on what you want, until each goal is a dream come true.

*"Those who dare
to fail miserably
can achieve greatly."*

-John F. Kennedy

ABOUT THE AUTHOR

Douglas Ellison is a medical researcher who specializes in natural healing methods. After reading hundreds of books and years of intensive study, he discovered the root cause of many chronic diseases. He also learned effective natural ways to prevent and cure them. His book will empower you with life changing knowledge that will help you create a healthier body, develop more self-control and achieve your goals.

To order more copies please go to:
healthrecoverysecrets.wordpress.com

or contact:
douglasjayellison@gmail.com

OTHER BOOKS
by Douglas J. Ellison

ADDICTION ANSWERS
A Practical Guide To
Creating Healthy Habits

INDEX

A
abstinance 176
acceptance 147
accomplishment 179
achieve 22, 25, 126, 145, 151, 157, 181, 187-191
acid 27, 31-33, 35, 68, 69, 99
acidic 17, 30, 68, 69, 169
acidosis 30, 53, 68, 72, 81, 83, 103
acids 68-70, 75, 83
acne 32
acupuncture 26, 89
addict 160, 175
addicted 130
addiction 4, 55, 116, 140, 159, 160, 162, 163, 166, 170-172, 175, 178, 192
addictive 102, 160, 162, 165, 168, 174, 175
addicts 160-162, 164
adrenaline 152, 153, 162, 163
aerobic 14, 16, 106
aholic 160
albicans 15, 17, 36, 118
alcohol 49, 57, 68-71, 78, 80, 82, 88, 97, 99, 116, 117, 160, 163-175, 183, 185
alcoholic 80, 83, 163, 166, 168-172
alcoholics 27, 117, 163, 166, 167, 169, 171-173, 175
alcoholism 166, 168, 171-173, 175
alkalize 28, 30, 104, 109, 169
alkalizing 27-29, 33, 52, 97, 99
Alkalosis 79
allergic 50, 56-58, 62, 99, 100
allergies 56, 171, 174
aluminum 54, 100
Alzheimer's 74
Amphetamines 55
anaerobic 14, 16, 71

cured 90, 113-115, 145

D

deficiencies 33, 50, 78, 93
deficiency 13, 14, 19-21, 25, 41, 60, 68, 81, 90
degenerative 26, 78, 79, 98, 100, 102
dehydrated 97
dehydration 28, 40, 67, 78, 81, 97, 99, 105
dementia 52, 78, 90, 97, 100, 184
demonic 120, 127-129
demons 126-131, 134, 139, 143, 153, 161, 178
denial 147, 148, 168
Dentists 75
dependency 99, 116, 159, 163, 168, 169, 175
depression 76, 84, 99, 115-118, 147, 148, 163
detox 27, 28, 33, 103, 169
diabetes 5, 24, 26, 50, 54, 76, 78, 82-84, 103
diagnose 2, 39, 85, 122
diarrhea 38, 40, 68, 6
diets 94, 117
digestion 137
digestive 38, 69, 79, 99, 100
diuretic 99
drugs 2-4, 7, 9-11, 13, 16, 20, 21, 23-25, 31, 41, 43, 48, 55-57,
67, 78, 80, 81, 87, 88, 103, 113-117, 119-122, 128, 130, 134,
150, 153, 160-164, 169, 173, 183
dyslexia 54

E

ebola 35, 40
echinacea 104
egomaniac 171
embolus 73
emotions 107, 115, 136-146, 149, 151, 154, 155, 157, 187
Emphysema 84
encephalitis 38
endometriosis 87
enema 26, 89
enzymes 29, 47, 48, 50, 79, 94, 96, 98, 99, 101
Ergotism 37

iodine 98
Irradiation 96
J
jaundice 20
joints 70, 76, 79, 80
juice 26, 27, 79, 88, 89, 169
juicing 27, 33
K
kale 27
kelp 98
kidney 20, 29, 68, 82, 83, 76, 97
L
lactose 99
Laetrile 27
Lalanne 92, 117
leprosy 11, 62, 63
lesions 53, 60, 74, 76
leukemia 14, 39, 56, 81
leukocytes 13
M
malignant 11
malnutrition 63, 67
MASTECTOMIES 87
medicine 3, 4, 7, 23, 28, 93, 95, 96
melanomas 12
Mendelsohn 18, 23, 45, 58, 85, 86
Merck 2, 3, 7, 9, 13, 19, 20, 35, 39, 40, 46, 53, 54, 72, 76
metabolic 53, 90, 102, 103
metabolism 103, 106
microorganisms 17, 36, 37, 68, 94, 123
mineral 26, 28, 33, 50, 68, 80, 90, 94
minerals 20, 27-29, 50, 75, 94, 97, 98, 100, 105, 109
molasses 100
mold 62, 85
molecular 47, 68
molecules 35, 77
moles 12, 31

www.ingramcontent.com/pod-product-compliance
Lightning Source LLC
Chambersburg PA
CBHW062143280526
45788CB00001B/289